Pediatric Inflammatory Bowel Disease

Editor

MARLA C. DUBINSKY

GASTROENTEROLOGY CLINICS OF NORTH AMERICA

www.gastro.theclinics.com

Consulting Editor
ALAN L. BUCHMAN

September 2023 • Volume 52 • Number 3

ELSEVIER

1600 John F. Kennedy Boulevard • Suite 1800 • Philadelphia, Pennsylvania, 19103-2899
http://www.theclinics.com

GASTROENTEROLOGY CLINICS OF NORTH AMERICA Volume 52, Number 3
September 2023 ISSN 0889-8553, ISBN-13: 978-0-443-18246-4

Editor: Kerry Holland
Developmental Editor: Hannah Almira Lopez

Gastroenterology Clinics of North America (ISSN 0889-8553) is published quarterly by Elsevier Inc., 360 Park Avenue South, New York, NY 10010-1710. Months of issue are March, June, September, and December. Business and Editorial Offices: 1600 John F. Kennedy Blvd., Suite 1800, Philadelphia, PA 19103-2899. Customer Service Office: 6277 Sea Harbor Drive, Orlando, FL 32887-4800. Periodicals postage paid at New York, NY and additional mailing offices. Subscription prices are $379.00 per year (US individuals), $100.00 per year (US students), $849.00 per year (US institutions), $407.00 per year (Canadian individuals), $100.00 per year (Canadian students), $1041.00 per year (Canadian institutions), $482.00 per year (international individuals), $220.00 per year (international students), and $1041.00 per year (international institutions). Foreign air speed delivery is included in all *Clinics* subscription prices. All prices are subject to change without notice. **POSTMASTER:** Send address changes to *Gastroenterology Clinics of North America*, Elsevier Health Sciences Division, Subscription Customer Service, 3251 Riverport Lane, Maryland Heights, MO 63043. **Telephone: 1-800-654-2452 (U.S. and Canada); 314-447-8871 (outside U.S. and Canada). Fax: 314-447-8029. E-mail: journalscustomerservice-usa@elsevier.com (for print support); journalsonlinesupport-usa@elsevier.com (for online support).**

Reprints. For copies of 100 or more, of articles in this publication, please contact the Commercial Reprints Department, Elsevier Inc., 360 Part Avenue South, New York, New York 10010-1710. Tel. 212-633-3874, Fax: 212-633-3820, E-mail: reprints@elsevier.com.

Gastroenterology Clinics of North America is also published in Italian by Il Pensiero Scientifico Editore, Rome, Italy; and in Portuguese by Interlivros Edicoes Ltda., Rua Commandante Coelho 1085, 21250 Cordovil, Rio de Janeiro, Brazil.

Gastroenterology Clinics of North America is covered in *MEDLINE/PubMed (Index Medicus), Excerpta Medica, Current Contents/Clinical Medicine, Science Citation Index, ISI/BIOMED,* and *BIOSIS.*

Contributors

CONSULTING EDITOR

ALAN L. BUCHMAN, MD, MSPH, FACP, FACN, FACG, AGAF
Professor of Clinical Surgery, Medical Director, Intestinal Rehabilitation and Transplant Center, The University of Illinois at Chicago/UI Health, Chicago, IL, USA

EDITOR

MARLA C. DUBINSKY, MD
Professor of Pediatrics and Medicine, Chief, Division of Pediatric GI and Nutrition, Co-director, Susan and Leonard Feinstein IBD Clinical Center, Director, Marie and Barry Lipman IBD Preconception and Pregnancy Clinic, Mount Sinai Kravis Children's Hospital, Icahn School of Medicine at Mount Sinai, New York, New York, USA

AUTHORS

LINDSEY ALBENBERG, DO
Attending Physician, Division of Gastroenterology, Hepatology, and Nutrition, Children's Hospital of Philadelphia, Assistant Professor of Pediatrics, Perelman School of Medicine, University of Pennsylvania, Philadelphia, Pennsylvania, USA

ERIC I. BENCHIMOL, MD, PhD
Professor of Paediatrics and Clinical Epidemiology, SickKids Inflammatory Bowel Disease Centre, Division of Gastroenterology, Hepatology and Nutrition, The Hospital for Sick Children (SickKids), Child Health Evaluative Sciences, SickKids Research Institute, ICES, Department of Paediatrics and Institute of Health Policy, Management and Evaluation, University of Toronto, Toronto, Ontario, Canada

JULIA DING, MD
Gastroenterology Fellow, Division of Gastroenterology and Hepatology, Boston University School of Medicine, Boston, Massachusetts, USA

MICHAEL TODD DOLINGER, MD, MBA
Assistant Professor of Pediatrics, Division of Pediatric Gastroenterology, Department of Pediatrics, Icahn School of Medicine at Mount Sinai, New York, New York, USA

LAURIE N. FISHMAN, MD
Gastroenterology Attending, Division of Gastroenterology and Nutrition, Boston Children's Hospital, Associate Professor in Pediatrics, Harvard Medical School, Boston, Massachusetts, USA

ANDREW GROSSMAN, MD
Professor of Clinical Pediatrics, Perelman School of Medicine, University of Pennsylvania, Children's Hospital of Philadelphia, Philadelphia, Pennsylvania, USA

JEFFREY S. HYAMS, MD
Mandell Braunstein Family Endowed Chair in Pediatric IBD, Head, Division of Digestive Diseases, Hepatology, and Nutrition, Connecticut Children's Medical Center, Hartford, Connecticut, USA; Professor of Pediatrics, University of Connecticut School of Medicine, Farmington, Connecticut, USA

LAURIE KEEFER, PhD
Professor of Medicine, Icahn School of Medicine at Mount Sinai, New York, New York, USA

RABIA KHAN, MD
Research Fellow, Division of Gastroenterology, SickKids Inflammatory Bowel Disease Centre, Hepatology and Nutrition, The Hospital for Sick Children (SickKids), Toronto, Ontario, Canada

SARA AHOLA KOHUT, PhD
Psychologist, Department of Gastroenterology, Hepatology, and Nutrition, The Hospital for Sick Children (SickKids), Toronto, Ontario, Canada

M. ELLEN KUENZIG, PhD
Senior Research Associate, SickKids Inflammatory Bowel Disease Centre, Division of Gastroenterology, Hepatology and Nutrition, The Hospital for Sick Children (SickKids), Child Health Evaluative Sciences, SickKids Research Institute, Toronto, Ontario, Canada

AARON M. LIPSKAR, MD
Associate Professor, Surgery and Pediatrics, Division of Pediatric Surgery, Cohen Children's Medical Center, Zucker School of Medicine at Hofstra/Northwell, New Hyde Park, New York, USA

PHILLIP MINAR, MD, MS
Associate Professor of Pediatrics, Division of Pediatric Gastroenterology, Hepatology and Nutrition, Cincinnati Children's Hospital Medical Center, Department of Pediatrics, University of Cincinnati School of Medicine, Cincinnati, Ohio, USA

ELANA B. MITCHEL, MD, MSCE
Assistant Professor of Clinical Pediatrics, Perelman School of Medicine, University of Pennsylvania, Children's Hospital of Philadelphia, Philadelphia, Pennsylvania, USA

ALEXANDER NASR, MD
Division of Pediatric Gastroenterology, Hepatology and Nutrition, Cincinnati Children's Hospital Medical Center, Cincinnati, Ohio, USA

JOEL R. ROSH, MD
Pediatric Gastroenterology, Professor of Pediatrics, Division of Pediatric Gastroenterology, Liver Disease, and Nutrition, Cohen Children's Medical Center of New York, Lake Success, New York, USA

RICHARD K. RUSSELL, MD, PhD
Consultant Paediatric Gastroenterologist, Department of Paediatric Gastroenterology, Royal Hospital for Children and Young People, Edinburgh, United Kingdom

ELIZABETH A. SPENCER, MD, MSc
Assistant Professor of Pediatrics, Division of Pediatric Gastroenterology and Nutrition, Department of Pediatrics, Icahn School of Medicine at Mount Sinai, New York, New York, USA

XIAOYI ZHANG, MD, PhD
Pediatric Gastroenterology, Assistant Professor of Clinical Pediatrics, Department of Pediatrics, Division of Gastroenterology, Hepatology and Nutrition, Indiana University, Indianapolis, Indiana, USA

Contents

Inflammatory bowel disease (IBD), including subtypes Crohn disease and ulcerative colitis, is a chronic inflammatory disorder most often diagnosed in young adulthood. The incidence and prevalence of pediatric-onset IBD is increasing globally. IBD is likely caused by an interplay of multiple environmental factors resulting in a dysregulated mucosal response to the commensal intestinal microbiota in genetically predisposed individuals. This article provides an overview of pediatric IBD epidemiology and environmental risk factors associated with its development, such as the Hygiene Hypothesis, air pollution, greenspace and blue space, neonatal factors, antibiotics, and diet.

Effectiveness of limited available therapies for pediatric inflammatory bowel disease has reached stagnation. Previous non-invasive monitoring strategies have relied upon cumbersome tools to evaluate clinical symptoms and biochemical markers that do not reflect endoscopic activity or respond quickly to treatments. Novel, patient-centric, and highly accurate, monitoring strategies with a focus on intestinal ultrasound for a direct, precise monitoring of activity to achieve disease modification are now possible. Ultimately, research on the optimal tight control monitoring strategies, individualized to each pediatric inflammatory bowel disease patient, are in development and offer a hope to potential therapeutic ceiling breakthrough on the horizon.

Despite the enlarging therapeutic armamentarium, IBD is still plagued by a therapeutic ceiling. Precision medicine, with the selection of the "rights," may present a solution, and this review will discuss the critical process of pairing the right patient with right therapy at the right time. Firstly, the review will discuss the shift to and evidence behind early effective therapy. Then, it delves into promising future strategies of patient profiling to identify a patients' biological pathway(s) and prognosis. Finally, the review lays out practical considerations that drive treatment selection, particularly the impact of the therapeutic sequence.

> Therapeutic options for the treatment of pediatric inflammatory bowel disease include aminosalicylates, enteral nutrition, corticosteroids, immunomodulators, biologics, and emerging small molecule agents. Infectious risk due to systemic immunosuppression should be mitigated by appropriate screening before therapy initiation. Rare but serious malignancies have been associated with thiopurine use alone and in combination with anti-tumor necrosis factor agents, often in the setting of a primary Epstein–Barr virus infection. Potential agent-specific adverse events such as cytopenias, hepatotoxicity, and nephrotoxicity warrant regular clinical and laboratory monitoring.

> The use of biologic therapies has changed the treatment landscape for children with inflammatory bowel disease. While the novel biologics have improved clinical outcomes, there remains a significant gap in achieving endoscopic remission, prolonged steroid-free remission, and drug durability. Contributing to this gap is the paucity of real-world pharmacokinetic studies in children and a failure to dose optimize therapy during induction. Emerging data from a pediatric clinical trial and several observational studies have shown that the combination of proactive therapeutic drug monitoring and achievement of early therapeutic concentrations is effective in achieving improved outcomes. The next steps will be to leverage these past studies to develop more innovative clinical trials to properly assess the safety and effectiveness of proactive therapeutic drug monitoring in children.

> The pathogenesis of inflammatory bowel disease (IBD) involves a complex interaction between genetics, immune response, and the environment. Epidemiologic associations between diet and development of IBD plus the ability of diet to modify the microbiota and modulate immune function have led to the hypothesis that diet can prevent and/or treat IBD. It is well established that the induction of remission and healing of the mucosa in Crohn's disease can be accomplished with exclusive enteral nutrition. Whole food-based alternatives such as the Crohn's disease exclusion diet have shown promising results.

> Surgery for children and adolescents with IBD is often thought of as a combination of a failure of medical management and the only option for the severe complications of the disease such as uncontrolled GI bleeding, perforation, fistulae, sepsis, and bowel obstruction. However, in CD, surgery can sometimes be an appropriate option to control disease progression, improve symptoms, allow children to get back on the growth curve,

and avoid the toxicities of prolonged use of steroids. In UC, the decision to operate is theoretically curative but the long-term options mandate either intestinal continuity with an ileal pouch or a lifelong ileostomy, both of which can have significant impacts in patients' quality of life.

The gap between available biologic and small molecule therapy for inflammatory bowel disease for children and adults remains large. At present only 2 anti-TNF agents are licensed for pediatric use compared with multiple other agents with different mechanisms of action being used in adults. The reasons are many but largely revolve around the inadequate acceptance of adult efficacy data to children, and the reluctance of industry to commit to early pediatric drug development for fear of inadequate return on investment. We suggest common sense steps that need to be taken to improve this situation.

Transition from pediatric to adult health care is a complex process that calls for complex interventions and collaboration between health care teams and families. However, many inflammatory bowel disease (IBD) clinical care teams do not have the resources to implement rigorous transition programs for youth. This review provides a description of the Resilience5: self-efficacy, disease acceptance, self-regulation, optimism, and social support. The Resilience5 represents teachable skills to support IBD self-management, offset disease interfering behaviors, and build resilience in adolescents and young adults transitioning to adult health care systems. These skills can also be encouraged and reinforced during routine IBD clinical care.

Patients with pediatric inflammatory bowel disease (pIBD) are at an increased risk for complications and comorbidities including infection, nutritional deficiencies, growth delay, bone disease, eye disease, malignancy, and psychologic disorders. Preventative health maintenance and monitoring is an important part to caring for patients with pIBD. Although practice is variable and published study within pIBD is limited, this article summarizes the important field of health-care maintenance in pIBD. A multidisciplinary approach, including the gastroenterologist provider, primary care provider, social worker, psychologist, as well as other subspecialists is necessary.

Health care transition from pediatric to adult care has been identified as a priority in the field of medicine, especially for those with chronic illnesses such as inflammatory bowel disease (IBD). Although there is no universally accepted model of preparing the pediatric patient for transfer to adult care, transition care is best accomplished in a structured and consistent manner. The authors highlight concepts for optimizing the transition of care for patients with IBD, which include setting expectations throughout adolescence with the gradual nurturing of self-management skills, preparing and assessing of readiness for transfer, and enacting a successful transfer to adult care.

GASTROENTEROLOGY
CLINICS OF NORTH AMERICA

THE CLINICS ARE AVAILABLE ONLINE!
Access your subscription at:
www.theclinics.com

Foreword

Can We all Be Champions?

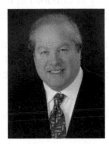

Alan L. Buchman, MD, MSPH, FACP, FACN, FACG, AGAF
Consulting Editor

Dr Marla Dubinsky has been a champion for kids (and adults) with inflammatory bowel disease (IBD) now for a couple of decades. She has assembled a group of international experts who address the particular nuances of IBD when it affects children, including the increasing number of afflicted kids and the growing recognition of the role personalized/precision medicine is starting to play. There are unique concerns when children have IBD, and they themselves have unique concerns as well. These are especially important in the area of growth and development—not just cognitive development but social/emotional, sexual, and athletic development as well. It is rare for children to have chronic diseases and thus it can be difficult for healthy children to interact with peers that have such medical problems, and equally challenging for those afflicted to have normal relations with their healthy friends. As Molly Roberts says in her song Champion, "You don't know what I've been through."

How can we be Champions? There clearly is a need to advance therapies more rapidly for children when they are readily available for adults. The FDA often requires studies in children, but this is problematic for pharmaceutical companies (just like pregnancy and the elderly) due largely to the high cost of insurance that evolves around potential safety issues. Although these are important concerns, there is an impediment to drug development in pediatrics despite the Pediatric Waiver.

Patients themselves can become Champions by understanding their disease, which requires a provider that understands that concept and can articulate it to their patients; to understand appropriate limitations and also how to develop countermeasures for those limitations such that the child controls their disease rather than the disease controlling the child.

We must all be cognizant of the fact that children are not just small adults. There are longer-term concerns from the diseases themselves as well as the treatments—or even running out of treatments for that matter. There are social issues that include the stigma of disease and potentially disease-limiting opportunities in education, social

Gastroenterol Clin N Am 52 (2023) xiii–xiv
https://doi.org/10.1016/j.gtc.2023.06.002
0889-8553/23/© 2023 Published by Elsevier Inc.

gastro.theclinics.com

and emotional development as well as physical activity. Diet is an important concern even in "healthy" children, let alone those that may have decreased nutrient absorption, decreased nutrient intake, and increased nutrient losses, notwithstanding potential treatment effects of specific diets. Intervention must be made early on to prevent growth abnormalities that may be irreversible.

We need to understand the ramifications of surgery in children in terms of nutrition as well as social development because once an organ is gone, there ain't no puttin' it back in.

Then, of course, there is the transition of care around age 18 to adult providers, although sometimes that transition is years or even decades later out of necessity.

"We need to be ready for the future when it calls out," as Molly Roberts sings. The future is now.

Alan L. Buchman, MD, MSPH, FACP, FACN, FACG, AGAF
Professor of Clinical Surgery
Medical Director
Intestinal Rehabilitation and Transplant Center
The University of Illinois at Chicago/UI Health
840 South Wood Street
Suite 402 (MC958)
Chicago, IL 60612, USA

E-mail address:
buchman@uic.edu

Preface

The Past, Present, and Future of Pediatric Inflammatory Bowel Disease

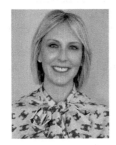

Marla C. Dubinsky, MD
Editor

Pediatric Inflammatory Bowel Disease (IBD) cases continue to rise globally, as does the demand for accurate and up-to-date information and education that pay special attention to the unique features and considerations for managing these patients. The state-of-the-art content in this special issue has been curated by leaders in the field in their respective areas of interest and expertise. This issue of *Gastroenterology Clinics of North America* highlights where we are in the field of IBD with a special emphasis on how the advances in the field apply to IBD diagnosed in childhood.

In addition to the changing epidemiology, the authors highlight the importance of precision medicine and treatment selection, including balancing the safety with the benefits of the therapy, the need for tight control monitoring, and adopting a treat-to-target strategy to optimize pediatric outcomes. Given the significant impact of uncontrolled inflammation and malnutrition on growth and development, the role of diet in IBD does often take a front seat in the overall management of pediatric IBD. Herein, we review the various ways diet can be integrated as sole therapy or in combination with other anti-inflammatory approaches. Not only is the impact of IBD on puberty a major differentiator from adult-onset IBD, so is the understanding on the role of resilience and self-management to help guide a successful transition plan to set our patients up for the successful transfer of care from a pediatric family-focused practice to that of a more autonomous and independent adult practice.

Despite the rapidly advancing therapeutic landscape for IBD, there remains significant delay to gaining regulatory approval for these same therapies in children, often resulting in off-label use without clear dosing guidance, and this review shares with the reader an expert's point of view and how to consider solving this problem, which has been in play since the late 1990s when infliximab, our first biologic therapy in

Gastroenterol Clin N Am 52 (2023) xv–xvi
https://doi.org/10.1016/j.gtc.2023.05.010
gastro.theclinics.com

IBD, was introduced. This special issue provides an accurate roadmap on how to approach the management of pediatric IBD and delivers some key insights into the future.

Marla C. Dubinsky, MD
Division of Pediatric GI and Nutrition
Susan and Leonard Feinstein IBD Clinical Center
Mount Sinai Kravis Children's Hospital
Icahn School of Medicine
Mount Sinai New York
17 East 102nd Street, Box 1134
New York, NY 10029, USA

E-mail address:
Marla.dubinsky@mssm.edu

Epidemiology of Pediatric Inflammatory Bowel Disease

Rabia Khan, MD[a], M. Ellen Kuenzig, PhD[a,b],
Eric I. Benchimol, MD, PhD[a,b,c,d],*

KEYWORDS

- Crohn disease • Ulcerative colitis • Incidence • Prevalence
- Environmental risk factors • Very early-onset IBD • Microbiome

KEY POINTS

- The worldwide incidence of pediatric IBD is increasing, and it is now routinely reported in regions with previously low prevalence.
- The age at which children are being diagnosed with IBD is decreasing, likely due to a combination of earlier disease onset, advanced diagnostic techniques, and improved access to specialist care.
- IBD is thought to result from a complex interaction between environmental and immune factors, likely mediated by the impact of these environmental exposures on the intestinal microbiome in genetically susceptible individuals.
- To understand the cause of IBD, particularly the increasing incidence of very early onset IBD, we must study populations where IBD is emerging using advanced epidemiologic methods.

INTRODUCTION

Inflammatory bowel disease (IBD) is a complex chronic multifactorial disorder that involves relapsing and remitting inflammation of the gastrointestinal tract. The most common subtypes are Crohn disease (CD) and ulcerative colitis (UC). IBD develops in genetically susceptible individuals who are exposed to specific environmental factors that may alter the intestinal microbiome, resulting in dysbiosis and immune dysregulation. It is suspected that genetic risk plays a greater role in pediatric-onset IBD, with some studies showing that higher polygenic risk scores and specific IBD risk

[a] SickKids Inflammatory Bowel Disease Centre, Division of Gastroenterology, Hepatology and Nutrition, The Hospital for Sick Children (SickKids), 555 University Avenue, Toronto, ON M5G 1X8, Canada; [b] Child Health Evaluative Sciences, SickKids Research Institute; [c] ICES, Toronto, Canada; [d] Department of Paediatrics and Institute of Health Policy, Management and Evaluation, University of Toronto, Toronto, Canada
* Corresponding author. Division of Gastroenterology, Hepatology and Nutrition, The Hospital for Sick Children, 555 University Avenue, Toronto, ON M5G 1X8.
E-mail address: eric.benchimol@sickkids.ca

Gastroenterol Clin N Am 52 (2023) 483–496
https://doi.org/10.1016/j.gtc.2023.05.001
0889-8553/23/© 2023 Elsevier Inc. All rights reserved.
gastro.theclinics.com

variants are associated with earlier disease onset[1,2] and a complicated disease course.[3] In children with very early onset IBD (VEOIBD), defined as disease onset at less than 6 years (y) of age, genetics are postulated to play an even greater role in the disease development, with more than 80 monogenic causes identified to date.[4] These mutations often cause primary immune deficiencies or epithelial barrier defects.

This article will explore our evolving knowledge of the epidemiology of IBD, including potential environmental causes, and differences across the age spectrum. In addition, we will explore the role of migration and ethnicity on the incidence of IBD, which may provide clues as to sociocultural elements, such as diet and environment, that may predispose some populations to the development of IBD.

THE EVOLVING EPIDEMIOLOGY OF PEDIATIRC INFLAMMATORY BOWEL DISEASE

There is a wide geographical variation in rates of pediatric IBD internationally (**Fig. 1**A).[5] Population-based studies report that both incidence and prevalence of IBD are highest in northern regions (Canada, Northern Europe, Northern United States, Israel, and New Zealand). Rates are lowest in Southern Europe, Asia, Africa, and the Middle East.[5] However, the data on the incidence and prevalence of pediatric IBD in many low and middle-income countries (LMICs) are sparse. Most data on the epidemiology of VEOIBD come from Western countries, where the overall incidence of IBD is highest (**Fig. 1**B).[5] Based on limited available research, the geographic variation in the incidence of VEOIBD seems to mirror that of pediatric IBD.

The incidence and prevalence of pediatric-onset IBD is increasing in most countries, continuing to increase in regions where incidence was already high and emerging in regions where it was previously not reported.[5,6] Kaplan and Windsor hypothesized that the evolution of IBD epidemiology follows 4 stages: (1) emergence, (2) acceleration in incidence, (3) compounding prevalence, and (4) prevalence equilibrium (**Fig. 2**).[7]

The incidence of adult-onset IBD has plateaued in many Western nations while its prevalence continues to climb,[6] consistent with the compounding prevalence stage. In contrast, the incidence of pediatric-onset IBD is still increasing in Western countries, suggesting pediatric IBD remains in the acceleration stage. Many LMICs remain in the emergence phase. However, some regions (eg, England[8]) have seen a stabilization in the incidence of pediatric IBD suggesting that we may soon reach the compounding prevalence stage for pediatric IBD in Western countries.[5]

The age at which children are diagnosed with IBD may be decreasing. However, age-specific trends in the incidence of IBD vary globally. In Canada, the incidence of VEOIBD is increasing at a faster rate than other age groups.[5] Similarly, the average age at IBD diagnosis among children in Israel has decreased.[9] In contrast, the incidence of VEOIBD has either decreased or remained stable in other regions, including Saudi Arabia, Finland, France, and the United Kingdom.[8] The countries with decreasing or stable incidence of VEOIBD have simultaneously reported increasing incidence rates among older children. Increases in incidence are likely multifactorial with changing environmental exposures (such as Westernization), increased awareness, access to specialist care and endoscopy, and improved imaging all contributing to increased risk or earlier diagnosis.[10,11] Prevalence of pediatric IBD is also increasing over time in all regions, across various age, and disease-specific groups.[12–17]

ETHNOCULTURAL BACKGROUND AND THE IMPACT OF MIGRATION

Studies describing ethnocultural differences in the epidemiology of IBD within a single geographic region can provide insight into the cause of IBD. An Israeli study reported increased in the prevalence of pediatric IBD, with prevalence increasing

A Pediatric-onset Inflammatory Bowel Disease

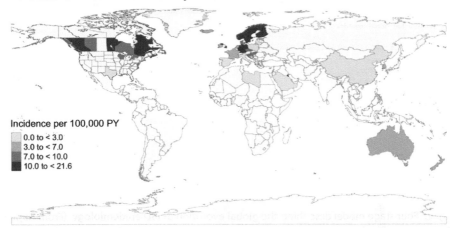

Incidence per 100,000 PY

- 0.0 to < 3.0
- 3.0 to < 7.0
- 7.0 to < 10.0
- 10.0 to < 21.6

B Very Early Onset Inflammatory Bowel Disease (VEOIBD)

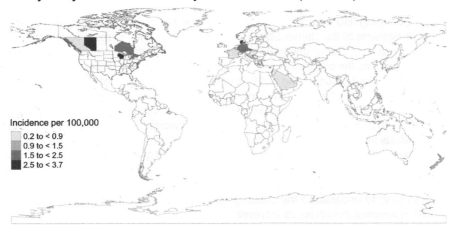

Incidence per 100,000

- 0.2 to < 0.9
- 0.9 to < 1.5
- 1.5 to < 2.5
- 2.5 to < 3.7

Fig. 1. Global incidence of (*A*) pediatric-onset IBD and (*B*) VEOIBD. (*From* Kuenzig ME, Fung SG, Marderfeld L, et al. Twenty-first Century Trends in the Global Epidemiology of Pediatric-Onset Inflammatory Bowel Disease: Systematic Review. Gastroenterology 2022;162:1147-1159; with permission.)

faster among Arabs than Jews.[9,18] Canadians of South Asian ethnicity have been demonstrated to have a higher incidence of IBD compared with Chinese Canadians, and a higher risk of UC compared with non-South Asian Canadians after adjusting for immigration status, implying that being born in Canada activated risk in people of South Asian origin.[19]

Studies of people migrating between areas with different background risk of developing IBD may provide valuable insights into the cause of IBD. People migrating from regions with low rates to those with high incidence of IBD are at lower risk of developing IBD compared with individuals born in high incidence regions.[20–22] However, the risk of developing IBD can vary by country of origin and age at diagnosis. A Canadian study reported a 14% (95% confidence interval [CI] 11%–18%) decrease in the

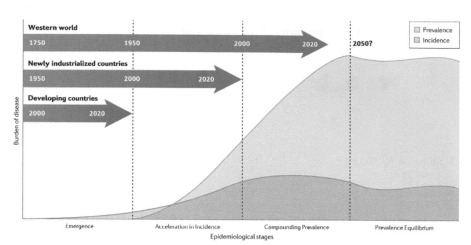

Fig. 2. Four-stage model describing the global evolution of IBD epidemiology. (*From* Kaplan GG, Windsor JW. The four epidemiological stages in the global evolution of inflammatory bowel disease. Nat Rev Gastroenterol Hepatol 2021;18:56-66; with permission.)

risk of developing IBD for every decade increase in the age at immigration.[22] Among Cuban immigrants to the United States, IBD presented earlier in more recent generations of migrants.[23] Some children of immigrants to Canada were at similar risk of developing IBD as the children of nonimmigrants; however, this depended on country of origin. Specifically, comparing children of mothers who were not immigrants, those born to parents emigrating from the Middle East, South Asia, Sub-Saharan Africa, and other Western nations had a similar risk of IBD, indicating the importance of early life exposure to the high-risk environment inherent in Canada.[21,22] The same is likely true for individuals immigrating to other Western nations.

Together, these findings suggest that ethnicity-related genetic disposition may protect certain individuals from IBD following migration. Studies describing changes in lifestyle and environmental exposures following immigration will become increasingly powerful tools to understand the cause of IBD as immigration from LMICs to Europe and North America continues to increase.

EARLY-LIFE ENVIRONMENTAL RISK FACTORS ASSOCIATED WITH INFLAMMATORY BOWEL DISEASE

The gut microbiome is different in children with IBD compared with heathy individuals.[24] Several of the environmental exposures associated with IBD likely act via their impact on the intestinal microbiome. Because the microbiome is established in early life, environmental exposures that coincide with this period may be more influential in the pathogenesis of pediatric-onset IBD. According to a systematic review and meta-analysis, 43 environmental exposures and lifestyle factors have been associated with IBD, with some of the strongest associations to pediatric IBD represented in **Fig. 3**.[25]

The Hygiene Hypothesis

Even before the evolution of our understanding of the gut microbiome, and the role the environment might play in microbiome composition, it was hypothesized that a lack of exposure to microorganisms detrimentally affects immune system development,

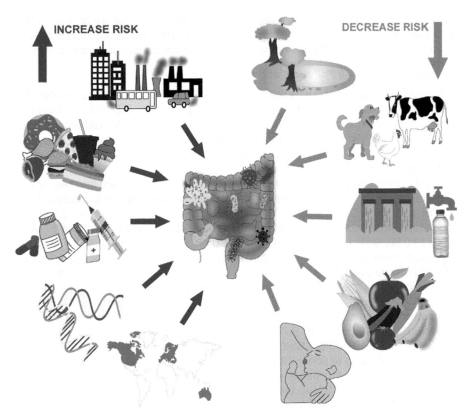

INCREASE RISK

DECREASE RISK

Fig. 3. Environmental factors that contribute to increased (left) or decreased (right) risk of IBD.

resulting in aberrant immune responses that may lead to immune-mediated inflammatory diseases including IBD. This concept is commonly referred to as the "Hygiene Hypothesis."

Indoor plumbing, household crowding, and exposure to pets or farm animals are often used as proxies for hygiene in studies evaluating the Hygiene Hypothesis. The heterogeneous findings of studies describing the associations between these factors and IBD preclude any concrete conclusions.

Studies describing the association between IBD and tap water are inconclusive.[26,27] However, the bacterial content of tap water has been associated with IBD. Increased exposure to coliform bacteria in tap water was associated with a decreased risk of UC (relative risk [RR] 0.99; 95% CI 0.98–1.00).[28] In an ecological study, the microbial composition of drinking water was associated with IBD.[29] In Africa, people who used bottled water as their primary drinking water source from 0 to 5 years of age had an increased odds of CD compared with those that primarily consumed, river, well, or dam water (odds ratio [OR] 2.1; 95% CI 1.2–4.0).[30]

Studies investigating the impact of household crowing, family size, and birth order on the risk of IBD have reached heterogenous conclusions. Some studies suggest large families and having older siblings decreases one's risk of IBD,[27,31,32] whereas other studies have failed to detect any association between household composition and IBD risk.[26,33–35]

Being exposed to pets or farm animals at a young age was associated with a decreased risk of IBD,[30,34,36] with some studies suggesting the association is specific to early life exposures.[36] These findings were consistent across geographic regions.

Urban Environment, Air Pollution, and Greenspace

Living in an urban area increases the risk of developing IBD[37] but the association between urban environment and IBD varies by age. A population-based Canadian study reported that the protective effect of living in a rural area was observed among those diagnosed during childhood and adolescence (<10 years: incidence rate ratio [IRR] 0.58, 95% CI 0.43–0.73; 10–18 years: IRR 0.72, 95% CI 0.64–0.81) but not during adulthood (IRR ranges 0.90–0.98).[38]

Air pollution may also be associated with IBD in an age-dependent manner. Among individuals aged 23 years or younger, NO_2 was associated with an increased risk of CD (OR 2.31, 95% CI 1.25–4.28).[39] In contrast, NO_2 and PM_{10} (but not SO_2) were associated with a decreased risk of CD among individuals between 44 and 57 years (NO_2: OR 0.56, 95% CI 0.33–0.95; PM_{10}: OR 0.48, 95% CI 0.29–0.80).[39] The redox-weighted oxidant capacity of air pollutants is associated with an increased risk of pediatric IBD (hazard ratio [HR] 1.08, 95% CI 1.01 to 1.16).[40] Translation studies suggest air pollution alters the intestinal microbiome in humans and mice,[41] resulting in dysbiosis.[42–44]

Both children and adults living near parks or in areas with ample trees are less likely to develop IBD (<18 years: HR 0.77, 95% CI 0.74–0.81; ≤10 years: HR 0.70, 95% CI 0.69–0.72; adults: HR 0.985, 95% CI 0.972–0.998).[45] In a prospective UK biobank study,[46] adults living in regions with more greenspace were also less likely to develop IBD. Each 5% increase in greenspace exposure was associated with a lower hazard of IBD (HR 0.978, 95% CI 0.966–0.990). Although blue space was not significantly associated with IBD when evaluated as a continuous variable (HR 0.978, 95% CI 0.873–1.095), it was protectively associated when comparing across tertiles (1 vs 3: HR 0.858, 95% CI 0.750–0.982; 2 vs 3: HR 0.785, 95% CI 0.685–0.899). Finally, regions classified as being in more natural environments were associated with lower risk of IBD (HR 0.977, 95% CI 0.966–0.988 for each 5% increase in natural environment).[46] Living in regions with a more natural environment may reduce stress, promote physical activity, and improve mental health. The combinations of these benefits, coupled with the benefits of nature on the gut microbiome, are probable mechanisms through which exposure to greenspace and blue space may reduce the risk of developing IBD.[46,47]

Cigarette Smoking

Although cigarette smoking is a well-established risk factor for adult-onset CD, no significant association between pediatric IBD and exposure to passive cigarette smoke has been reported in the literature, including when assessing prenatal exposure (CD: OR 1.10, 95% CI 0.67–1.80; UC: OR 1.11, 95% CI 0.63–1.97) or during early childhood (CD: OR 1.10, 95% CI 0.92–1.30; UC: OR 1.01, 95% CI 0.85–1.20).[48]

Mode of Delivery

Mode of birth affects the development of intestinal microbiota[49] because vaginal birth exposes infants to the maternal vaginal microbiome on delivery. Infants delivered by Cesarean section (C-section) harbor a different microbiome; however, it has been postulated that these changes may disappear by 6 weeks of life.[50] Nevertheless, C-section delivery has been thought to be associated with immune-medicated inflammatory diseases such as IBD.[51,52] However, meta-analyses have not demonstrated a significant association between C-section and the subsequent risk of IBD.[53,54]

Infant Feeding

The neonatal microbiome profile is influenced by feeding, and the literature has pointed to marked differences in the microbiome between children who are breastfed or formula-fed.[49] In infants who are not breastfed, the microbiome attains stability (or "maturity") at 3 months of age, whereas maturity is not reached until 12 months of age in those who are continuously breastfed, which plays a crucial role in promoting healthy microbiome.[55] Systematic reviews have reported a protective association between breastfeeding and pediatric-onset IBD, demonstrating a dose-dependent association.[56] There is a strong protective association when an infant is breastfed for at least 12 months with CD (OR 0.20, 95% CI 0.08–0.50) and UC (OR 0.21, 95% CI 0.10–0.43).[57]

Antibiotics Exposure

Antibiotics have an impactful effect on the microbiome and potentially contribute to dysbiosis with transiently decreased bacterial diversity, causing immune dysregulation. Early-life antibiotic exposure may have a long-lasting impact on the microbiome[58] because the first years of life are associated with the maturation period for infant's gut microbiome and enteric immune system.[59] Accordingly, antibiotic exposure during childhood has been associated with an increased risk of IBD, with antibiotics during the first year of life most strongly associated with later development of IBD.[60] As reported in a population-based study from England, a dose–response effect was noted with greater than 2 antibiotic courses more strongly associated with IBD. This study also found that the timing of antibiotic exposure is important; children receiving antibiotics before 1 year had the greatest increased risk (HR 5.51, 95% CI 1.66–18.28) compared with children receiving antibiotics before 5 years (HR 2.26, 95% CI 1.61–4.25) or 15 years (HR 1.57, 95% CI 1.35–1.84).[61] These findings suggest that childhood antibiotic exposure is most strongly associated with IBD at younger ages. Another meta-analysis demonstrated that the association among early-life antibiotics use was specific to CD (OR 2.75, 95% CI 1.72–4.38), and there was no association between early-life antibiotic use and UC (OR 1.08, 95% CI 0.91–1.27).[62]

Vaccinations

A systematic review and meta-analysis found no association among 7 childhood vaccines (BCG, diphtheria, tetanus, smallpox, poliomyelitis, measles-containing vaccines, and influenza vaccine) and the risk of developing IBD.[63] A small study of 70 children from Southeast Asia found that being vaccinated for rotavirus reduced the odds of developing IBD, an association present for both CD (OR 0.28, 95% CI 0.08–0.99) and UC (OR 0.42, 95% CI 0.11–1.56).[64] This contradicts a study from the United States of 333 patients diagnosed with IBD less than 10 years, which found no association with rotavirus vaccine (OR 0.72, 95% CI; 0.19–2.65).[65] At the time of writing, no studies have evaluated the association between COVID-19 vaccines and the risk of IBD. Annual influenza vaccination was not associated with flares of IBD.[66]

DIET

Although it is probable that diet affects the intestinal immunity, likely through modulation of the gut microbiome, studying the potential role of diet as a contributor to development of IBD is very challenging. The Westernization of local diets in LMICs is likely to contribute to the increasing incidence of IBD in those countries, although this is difficult to study in uncontrolled studies. However, some observational studies have demonstrated associations between dietary patterns and risk of IBD. Systematic reviews have also reported an increased risk of IBD with diets that are high in animal protein and saturated fat and low in fiber, fruits, and vegetables.[35,67,68]

Protein, Fat, and Carbohydrate Intake

A meta-analysis found no association between the risk of CD and intake of carbohydrates (RR 0.991, 95% CI 0.978–1.004), fats (RR 1.018, 95% CI 0.969–1.069), or protein (RR 1.029, 95% CI 0.955–1.109).[69] All RRs were expressed per 10 g increase in daily consumption. However, a large prospective European study concluded that red meat intake was associated with UC (HR 1.40, 95% CI 0.99–1.98) but found no association between food source and CD, including processed meat, fish, shellfish, eggs, and poultry.[70]

The data on dietary fat intake are less consistent. Many studies have failed to identify an association between overall fat intake and risk of CD and UC. An analysis from European Prospective Cohort Into Cancer (EPIC) Cohort demonstrated that higher fat intake, especially with arachidonic acid content, was associated with an increased risk of UC.[71] In contrast, dietary n-3 polyunsaturated fatty acid was protective against UC.[72] Studies of the association between carbohydrate intake and risk of CD and UC have not demonstrated consistent findings.

Fiber, Fruit, and Vegetable Intake

Fiber has an influence on the gut microbiome, particularly augmenting butyrate production (with its anti-inflammatory effect). A meta-analysis found that the intake of dietary fiber in the form of consumption of fruits and vegetables may be associated with the risk of IBD. Vegetable intake was associated with a lower risk of UC (OR 0.71, 95% CI 0.58–0.88) but not CD (OR 0.66, 95% CI 0.40–1.09), although statistical power may have played a role.[73] The protective effect has been hypothesized due to high fiber, micronutrients (vitamins C, E, and folate) and/or phytochemicals in fruits and vegetables that have been shown to reduce mucosal inflammation and maintain intestinal barrier function.[73] In the aforementioned meta-analysis, subgroup analyses showed a significant association for studies carried out in Europe (OR 0.36; 95% CI 0.23–0.57) but not in Asia (OR 1.00, 95% CI 0.50–2.03), emphasizing regional, geographic, or ethnocultural differences. This was similarly demonstrated in the differential effect of the Mediterranean diet on the gut microbiome in North American compared with other populations in a prospective cohort study.[74] The source of dietary fiber may also be very important. Various fiber subtypes have shown anti-inflammatory benefits. Fiber intake from fruits and vegetables (soluble fiber) has been found to be protective against CD, whereas insoluble fiber intake from such as cereals, whole grain, and legumes is not associated with CD or UC.[75]

Food Additives

Food additives include preservatives, artificial sweeteners, flavor enhancers, emulsifiers, thickeners, and other natural or chemical substances that prolong food storage and enrich nutrients. Commonly found in ultraprocessed foods, these additives can promote proinflammatory intestinal microbiota, disrupt mucus architecture, increase intestinal permeability, activate inflammatory pathways, and disrupt the cell cycle.[76–78] A prospective cohort study of adults from 21 countries found that ultraprocessed food was associated with higher risk of IBD ($\geq$5 servings per day: HR 1.82, 95% CI 1.22–2.72; 1–4 servings per day: HR 1.67, 95% CI 1.18–2.37).[79] In mice, dietary emulsifiers induced stress and low-grade inflammation by disrupting the microbiome and increased the susceptibility of developing experimental colitis.[78]

Other Micronutrients

Nutritional deficiencies have not been consistently associated with IBD. However, a meta-analysis found higher rates of vitamin D deficiency compared with controls in people with IBD (OR 1.64, 95% CI 1.30–2.08) and UC (OR 2.28, 95% CI 1.18–4.41).[80] A recent Danish study found that prenatal exposure to vitamin D from food fortification of margarine may protect against the development of IBD at an age of less than 30 years (OR 0.87, 95% CI 0.79–0.95).[81] However, as with most observational research, these studies could not determine whether vitamin D deficiency resulted in IBD development, was the result of active inflammation, or was a confounder.

DISCUSSION

The growing global burden of pediatric IBD, particularly VEOIBD, presents us with an important opportunity for research. Several of the environmental risk factors identified seem to be age-specific: smoking may be specific to adults, whereas air pollution and the urban environment may be specific to children and young adults. It is conceivable that the impact of specific environmental exposures may be even greater in young children, as is seen with the protectiveness of rurality and greenspace, and risk of early-life antibiotics. As more children develop IBD, both in Western countries and LMICs, we must aim to better understand the complex interaction between environmental exposures and the gut microbiome in genetically susceptible individuals from diverse ethnocultural backgrounds—including how different combinations of environmental exposures result in different IBD phenotypes (age at diagnosis, type of IBD, disease behavior and location in CD, and disease extent in UC).

SUMMARY

The burden of IBD is increasing globally and our understanding of the epidemiology of pediatric IBD has evolved over the years. However, we still have a limited understanding of the rates of IBD in children in LMICs, and how environmental factors influence IBD pathogenesis. Because children are exposed to fewer environmental risk factors during the course of their short lives compared with adults, they present us with an opportunity to better delineate the role of these environmental factors in the pathophysiology of IBD. However, only by studying the increasing tide of pediatric IBD in LMICs, ethnocultural differences in the interaction between exposures and genetics, and the effect of migration from low-income to high-income countries can we fully understand the epidemiology of IBD in children.

CLINICS CARE POINTS

- As the prevalence of IBD continues to increase around the world, primary care providers and gastroenterologists should be aware of the growing number of children with IBD. Because early diagnosis is critical to the long-term outcomes of children with IBD, identifying and treating these children as early as possible is vital.
- Health systems should be prepared for the growing number of children with IBD, providing adequate access to high-quality specialist care, endoscopy, cross-sectional imaging and IBD treatments.

- Prospective cohort studies of children living in areas where IBD is emerging, particularly in LMICs, are urgently needed so that we can gain a better understanding of the impact of economic development, Westernization, and environmental factors on the risk of IBD. This will allow us to understand disease pathogenesis, develop better treatments, and potentially stem the increase of new diagnoses through prevention.

DISCLOSURE

E.I. Benchimol holds the Northbridge Financial Corporation Chair in Inflammatory Bowel Disease, a joint Hospital-University Chair between the University of Toronto, The Hospital for Sick Children, and the SickKids Foundation. He has acted as a consultant for the Dairy Farmers of Ontario and McKesson Canada for matters unrelated to medications used to treat IBD.

REFERENCES

1. Hubenthal M, Loscher BS, Erdmann J, et al. Current Developments of Clinical Sequencing and the Clinical Utility of Polygenic Risk Scores in Inflammatory Diseases. Front Immunol 2020;11:577677.
2. Kuenzig ME, Yim J, Coward S, et al. The NOD2-Smoking Interaction in Crohn's Disease is likely Specific to the 1007fs Mutation and may be Explained by Age at Diagnosis: A Meta-Analysis and Case-Only Study. EBioMedicine 2017;21: 188–96.
3. Zheng HB, de la Morena MT, Suskind DL. The Growing Need to Understand Very Early Onset Inflammatory Bowel Disease. Front Immunol 2021;12:675186.
4. Uhlig HH, Schwerd T, Koletzko S, et al. The diagnostic approach to monogenic very early onset inflammatory bowel disease. Gastroenterology 2014;147: 990–1007 e3.
5. Kuenzig ME, Fung SG, Marderfeld L, et al. Twenty-first Century Trends in the Global Epidemiology of Pediatric-Onset Inflammatory Bowel Disease: Systematic Review. Gastroenterology 2022;162:1147–1159 e4.
6. Ng SC, Shi HY, Hamidi N, et al. Worldwide incidence and prevalence of inflammatory bowel disease in the 21st century: a systematic review of population-based studies. Lancet 2017;390:2769–78.
7. Kaplan GG, Windsor JW. The four epidemiological stages in the global evolution of inflammatory bowel disease. Nat Rev Gastroenterol Hepatol 2021;18:56–66.
8. Ashton JJ, Cullen M, Afzal NA, et al. Is the incidence of paediatric inflammatory bowel disease still increasing? Arch Dis Child 2018;103:1093–4.
9. Stulman MY, Asayag N, Focht G, et al. Epidemiology of Inflammatory Bowel Diseases in Israel: A Nationwide Epi-Israeli IBD Research Nucleus Study. Inflamm Bowel Dis 2021;27:1784–94.
10. Benchimol EI, Guttmann A, To T, et al. Changes to surgical and hospitalization rates of pediatric inflammatory bowel disease in Ontario, Canada (1994-2007). Inflamm Bowel Dis 2011;17:2153–61.
11. Carroll MW, Kuenzig ME, Mack DR, et al. The Impact of Inflammatory Bowel Disease in Canada 2018: Children and Adolescents with IBD. J Can Assoc Gastroenterol 2019;2:S49–67.
12. Benchimol EI, Bernstein CN, Bitton A, et al. Trends in Epidemiology of Pediatric Inflammatory Bowel Disease in Canada: Distributed Network Analysis of Multiple Population-Based Provincial Health Administrative Databases. Am J Gastroenterol 2017;112:1120–34.

13. Chan JM, Carroll MW, Smyth M, et al. Comparing Health Administrative and Clinical Registry Data: Trends in Incidence and Prevalence of Pediatric Inflammatory Bowel Disease in British Columbia. Clin Epidemiol 2021;13:81–90.

14. Benchimol EI, Manuel DG, Guttmann A, et al. Changing age demographics of inflammatory bowel disease in Ontario, Canada: a population-based cohort study of epidemiology trends. Inflamm Bowel Dis 2014;20:1761–9.

15. Ishige T, Tomomasa T, Hatori R, et al. Temporal Trend of Pediatric Inflammatory Bowel Disease: Analysis of National Registry Data 2004 to 2013 in Japan. J Pediatr Gastroenterol Nutr 2017;65:e80–2.

16. El-Matary W, Moroz SP, Bernstein CN. Inflammatory bowel disease in children of Manitoba: 30 years' experience of a tertiary center. J Pediatr Gastroenterol Nutr 2014;59:763–6.

17. Coward S, Clement F, Benchimol EI, et al. Past and Future Burden of Inflammatory Bowel Diseases Based on Modeling of Population-Based Data. Gastroenterology 2019;156:1345–53.e4.

18. Ghersin I, Khteeb N, Katz LH, et al. Trends in the epidemiology of inflammatory bowel disease among Jewish Israeli adolescents: a population-based study. Aliment Pharmacol Ther 2019;49:556–63.

19. Dhaliwal J, Tuna M, Shah BR, et al. Incidence of Inflammatory Bowel Disease in South Asian and Chinese People: A Population-Based Cohort Study from Ontario, Canada. Clin Epidemiol 2021;13:1109–18.

20. Agrawal M, Corn G, Shrestha S, et al. Inflammatory bowel diseases among first-generation and second-generation immigrants in Denmark: a population-based cohort study. Gut 2021;70:1037–43.

21. Li X, Sundquist J, Hemminki K, et al. Risk of inflammatory bowel disease in first- and second-generation immigrants in Sweden: a nationwide follow-up study. Inflamm Bowel Dis 2011;17:1784–91.

22. Benchimol EI, Mack DR, Guttmann A, et al. Inflammatory bowel disease in immigrants to Canada and their children: a population-based cohort study. Am J Gastroenterol 2015;110:553–63.

23. Damas OM, Avalos DJ, Palacio AM, et al. Inflammatory bowel disease is presenting sooner after immigration in more recent US immigrants from Cuba. Aliment Pharmacol Ther 2017;46:303–9.

24. Fitzgerald RS, Sanderson IR, Claesson MJ. Paediatric Inflammatory Bowel Disease and its Relationship with the Microbiome. Microb Ecol 2021;82:833–44.

25. Piovani D, Danese S, Peyrin-Biroulet L, et al. Environmental Risk Factors for Inflammatory Bowel Diseases: An Umbrella Review of Meta-analyses. Gastroenterology 2019;157:647–659 e4.

26. Baron S, Turck D, Leplat C, et al. Environmental risk factors in paediatric inflammatory bowel diseases: a population based case control study. Gut 2005;54:357–63.

27. Hampe J, Heymann K, Krawczak M, et al. Association of inflammatory bowel disease with indicators for childhood antigen and infection exposure. Int J Colorectal Dis 2003;18:413–7.

28. Aamodt G, Bukholm G, Jahnsen J, et al. The association between water supply and inflammatory bowel disease based on a 1990-1993 cohort study in southeastern Norway. Am J Epidemiol 2008;168:1065–72.

29. Forbes JD, Van Domselaar G, Sargent M, et al. Microbiome profiling of drinking water in relation to incidence of inflammatory bowel disease. Can J Microbiol 2016;62:781–93.

30. Basson A, Swart R, Jordaan E, et al. The association between childhood environmental exposures and the subsequent development of Crohn's disease in the Western Cape, South Africa. PLoS One 2014;9:e115492.

31. Bernstein CN, Rawsthorne P, Cheang M, et al. A population-based case control study of potential risk factors for IBD. Am J Gastroenterol 2006;101:993–1002.

32. Klement E, Lysy J, Hoshen M, et al. Childhood hygiene is associated with the risk for inflammatory bowel disease: a population-based study. Am J Gastroenterol 2008;103:1775–82.

33. Montgomery SM, Lambe M, Wakefield AJ, et al. Siblings and the risk of inflammatory bowel disease. Scand J Gastroenterol 2002;37:1301–8.

34. Strisciuglio C, Giugliano F, Martinelli M, et al. Impact of Environmental and Familial Factors in a Cohort of Pediatric Patients With Inflammatory Bowel Disease. J Pediatr Gastroenterol Nutr 2017;64:569–74.

35. Aujnarain A, Mack DR, Benchimol EI. The role of the environment in the development of pediatric inflammatory bowel disease. Curr Gastroenterol Rep 2013; 15:326.

36. Radon K, Windstetter D, Poluda AL, et al. Contact with farm animals in early life and juvenile inflammatory bowel disease: a case-control study. Pediatrics 2007; 120:354–61.

37. Soon IS, Molodecky NA, Rabi DM, et al. The relationship between urban environment and the inflammatory bowel diseases: a systematic review and meta-analysis. BMC Gastroenterol 2012;12:51.

38. Benchimol EI, Kaplan GG, Otley AR, et al. Rural and Urban Residence During Early Life is Associated with Risk of Inflammatory Bowel Disease: A Population-Based Inception and Birth Cohort Study. Am J Gastroenterol 2017;112:1412–22.

39. Kaplan GG, Hubbard J, Korzenik J, et al. The inflammatory bowel diseases and ambient air pollution: a novel association. Am J Gastroenterol 2010;105:2412–9.

40. Elten M, Benchimol EI, Fell DB, et al. Ambient air pollution and the risk of pediatric-onset inflammatory bowel disease: A population-based cohort study. Environ Int 2020;138:105676.

41. Fouladi F, Bailey MJ, Patterson WB, et al. Air pollution exposure is associated with the gut microbiome as revealed by shotgun metagenomic sequencing. Environ Int 2020;138:105604.

42. Vignal C, Guilloteau E, Gower-Rousseau C, et al. Review article: Epidemiological and animal evidence for the role of air pollution in intestinal diseases. Sci Total Environ 2021;757:143718.

43. Salim SY, Jovel J, Wine E, et al. Exposure to ingested airborne pollutant particulate matter increases mucosal exposure to bacteria and induces early onset of inflammation in neonatal IL-10-deficient mice. Inflamm Bowel Dis 2014;20: 1129–38.

44. Kish L, Hotte N, Kaplan GG, et al. Environmental particulate matter induces murine intestinal inflammatory responses and alters the gut microbiome. PLoS One 2013;8:e62220.

45. Elten M, Benchimol EI, Fell DB, et al. Residential Greenspace in Childhood Reduces Risk of Pediatric Inflammatory Bowel Disease: A Population-Based Cohort Study. Am J Gastroenterol 2021;116:347–53.

46. Zhang Z, Chen L, Qian ZM, et al. Residential green and blue space associated with lower risk of adult-onset inflammatory bowel disease: Findings from a large prospective cohort study. Environ Int 2022;160:107084.

47. Markevych I, Schoierer J, Hartig T, et al. Exploring pathways linking greenspace to health: Theoretical and methodological guidance. Environ Res 2017;158: 301–17.
48. Jones DT, Osterman MT, Bewtra M, et al. Passive smoking and inflammatory bowel disease: a meta-analysis. Am J Gastroenterol 2008;103:2382–93.
49. Azad MB, Konya T, Maughan H, et al. Gut microbiota of healthy Canadian infants: profiles by mode of delivery and infant diet at 4 months. CMAJ (Can Med Assoc J) 2013;185:385–94.
50. Chu DM, Ma J, Prince AL, et al. Maturation of the infant microbiome community structure and function across multiple body sites and in relation to mode of delivery. Nat Med 2017;23:314–26.
51. Sevelsted A, Stokholm J, Bonnelykke K, et al. Cesarean section and chronic immune disorders. Pediatrics 2015;135:e92–8.
52. Frias Gomes C, Narula N, Morao B, et al. Mode of Delivery Does Not Affect the Risk of Inflammatory Bowel Disease. Dig Dis Sci 2021;66:398–407.
53. Li Y, Tian Y, Zhu W, et al. Cesarean delivery and risk of inflammatory bowel disease: a systematic review and meta-analysis. Scand J Gastroenterol 2014;49: 834–44.
54. Bruce A, Black M, Bhattacharya S. Mode of delivery and risk of inflammatory bowel disease in the offspring: systematic review and meta-analysis of observational studies. Inflamm Bowel Dis 2014;20:1217–26.
55. Fehr K, Moossavi S, Sbihi H, et al. Breastmilk Feeding Practices Are Associated with the Co-Occurrence of Bacteria in Mothers' Milk and the Infant Gut: the CHILD Cohort Study. Cell Host Microbe 2020;28:285–297 e4.
56. Barclay AR, Russell RK, Wilson ML, et al. Systematic review: the role of breast-feeding in the development of pediatric inflammatory bowel disease. J Pediatr 2009;155:421–6.
57. Xu L, Lochhead P, Ko Y, et al. Systematic review with meta-analysis: breastfeeding and the risk of Crohn's disease and ulcerative colitis. Aliment Pharmacol Ther 2017;46:780–9.
58. Gevers D, Kugathasan S, Denson LA, et al. The treatment-naive microbiome in new-onset Crohn's disease. Cell Host Microbe 2014;15:382–92.
59. Shaw SY, Blanchard JF, Bernstein CN. Association between the use of antibiotics in the first year of life and pediatric inflammatory bowel disease. Am J Gastroenterol 2010;105:2687–92.
60. Kamphorst K, Van Daele E, Vlieger AM, et al. Early life antibiotics and childhood gastrointestinal disorders: a systematic review. BMJ Paediatr Open 2021;5: e001028.
61. Kronman MP, Zaoutis TE, Haynes K, et al. Antibiotic exposure and IBD development among children: a population-based cohort study. Pediatrics 2012;130: e794–803.
62. Ungaro R, Bernstein CN, Gearry R, et al. Antibiotics associated with increased risk of new-onset Crohn's disease but not ulcerative colitis: a meta-analysis. Am J Gastroenterol 2014;109:1728–38.
63. Pineton de Chambrun G, Dauchet L, Gower-Rousseau C, et al. Vaccination and Risk for Developing Inflammatory Bowel Disease: A Meta-Analysis of Case-Control and Cohort Studies. Clin Gastroenterol Hepatol 2015;13:1405–14015.e1 [quiz: e130].
64. Lee WS, Song ZL, Wong SY, et al. Environmental risk factors for inflammatory bowel disease: A case control study in Southeast Asian children. J Paediatr Child Health 2022;58:782–90.

65. Liles E, Irving SA, Dandamudi P, et al. Incidence of pediatric inflammatory bowel disease within the Vaccine Safety Datalink network and evaluation of association with rotavirus vaccination. Vaccine 2021;39:3614–20.
66. Benchimol EI, Hawken S, Kwong JC, et al. Safety and utilization of influenza immunization in children with inflammatory bowel disease. Pediatrics 2013;131: e1811–20.
67. Wark G, Samocha-Bonet D, Ghaly S, et al. The Role of Diet in the Pathogenesis and Management of Inflammatory Bowel Disease: A Review. Nutrients 2020; 13:135.
68. Andersen V, Olsen A, Carbonnel F, et al. Diet and risk of inflammatory bowel disease. Dig Liver Dis 2012;44:185–94.
69. Zeng L, Hu S, Chen P, et al. Macronutrient Intake and Risk of Crohn's Disease: Systematic Review and Dose-Response Meta-Analysis of Epidemiological Studies. Nutrients 2017;9:500.
70. Dong C, Chan SSM, Jantchou P, et al. Meat Intake Is Associated with a Higher Risk of Ulcerative Colitis in a Large European Prospective Cohort Studyo. J Crohns Colitis 2022;16:1187–96.
71. de Silva PS, Olsen A, Christensen J, et al. An association between dietary arachidonic acid, measured in adipose tissue, and ulcerative colitis. Gastroenterology 2010;139:1912–7.
72. John S, Luben R, Shrestha SS, et al. Dietary n-3 polyunsaturated fatty acids and the aetiology of ulcerative colitis: a UK prospective cohort study. Eur J Gastroenterol Hepatol 2010;22:602–6.
73. Li F, Liu X, Wang W, et al. Consumption of vegetables and fruit and the risk of inflammatory bowel disease: a meta-analysis. Eur J Gastroenterol Hepatol 2015;27: 623–30.
74. Turpin W, Dong M, Sasson G, et al. Mediterranean-Like Dietary Pattern Associations With Gut Microbiome Composition and Subclinical Gastrointestinal Inflammation. Gastroenterology 2022;163:685–98.
75. Armstrong H, Mander I, Zhang Z, et al. Not All Fibers Are Born Equal; Variable Response to Dietary Fiber Subtypes in IBD. Front Pediatr 2020;8:620189.
76. Viennois E, Bretin A, Dube PE, et al. Dietary Emulsifiers Directly Impact Adherent-Invasive E. coli Gene Expression to Drive Chronic Intestinal Inflammation. Cell Rep 2020;33:108229.
77. Bancil AS, Sandall AM, Rossi M, et al. Food Additive Emulsifiers and Their Impact on Gut Microbiome, Permeability, and Inflammation: Mechanistic Insights in Inflammatory Bowel Disease. J Crohns Colitis 2021;15:1068–79.
78. Laudisi F, Stolfi C, Monteleone G. Impact of Food Additives on Gut Homeostasis. Nutrients 2019;11:2334.
79. Narula N, Wong ECL, Dehghan M, et al. Association of ultra-processed food intake with risk of inflammatory bowel disease: prospective cohort study. BMJ 2021;374:n1554.
80. Del Pinto R, Pietropaoli D, Chandar AK, et al. Association Between Inflammatory Bowel Disease and Vitamin D Deficiency: A Systematic Review and Meta-analysis. Inflamm Bowel Dis 2015;21:2708–17.
81. Duus KS, Moos C, Frederiksen P, et al. Prenatal and Early Life Exposure to the Danish Mandatory Vitamin D Fortification Policy Might Prevent Inflammatory Bowel Disease Later in Life: A Societal Experiment. Nutrients 2021;13:1367.

The Role of Noninvasive Surrogates of Inflammation in Monitoring Pediatric Inflammatory Bowel Diseases
The Old and the New

Michael Todd Dolinger, MD, MBA*

KEYWORDS

- Tight-control • Intestinal ultrasound • Magnetic resonance enterography
- C-reactive protein

KEY POINTS

- Relying on clinical symptoms and biochemical is not accurate to monitor endoscopic inflammatory bowel disease activity.
- Use of non-invasive, reliable, patient-centric monitoring tools as surrogates of inflammation is even more critical in children whose parents are reluctant to have them undergo sedation for a colonoscopy.
- Intestinal ultrasound is an emerging, underutilized, non-invasive, point-of-care tool to monitor inflammatory bowel disease activity in children.
- Tight control monitoring using a combination of clinical scores, CRP, fecal calprotectin, and intestinal ultrasound to reach deep healing evaluated by MRE and wireless capsule endoscopy can be a patient-centric strategy to achieve disease modification and alter inflammatory bowel disease natural history.

INTRODUCTION

Crohn's disease and ulcerative colitis are progressive, relapsing and remitting, inflammatory bowel diseases (IBD) that lead to chronic damage often resulting in complications and surgery.[1,2] Consequently, pediatric-onset IBDs are more effectual than that of their adult counterparts, more aggressive, severe, and unstable in disease course, location, and nature over a longer duration associated with increased rates

Division of Pediatric Gastroenterology, Department of Pediatrics, Icahn School of Medicine at Mount Sinai, New York, NY, USA
* Icahn School of Medicine at Mount Sinai, Susan and Leonard Feinstein Inflammatory Bowel Disease Center, 17 East 102nd Street, 5th Floor, New York, NY 10029.
E-mail address: Michael.Dolinger@mssm.edu
Twitter: @DrMikeDolinger (M.T.D.)

Gastroenterol Clin N Am 52 (2023) 497–515
https://doi.org/10.1016/j.gtc.2023.05.003
0889-8553/23/© 2023 Elsevier Inc. All rights reserved.

of hospitalization and surgery.[3–8] Due to both the longevity and severity of pediatric IBDs, a treatment approach with a goal of healing the bowel may be even more important than in adults to achieve disease modification and alter long-term natural history. Despite a lack of prospective data, current expert consensus is to achieve a target of mucosal healing in children with IBD through the use of tight control monitoring to catch disease drift, thus preventing chronic bowel damage and subsequent complications from occurring.[9,10] Further, pediatric Crohn's disease present a unique challenge for non-invasive monitoring, presenting with extensive small bowel disease, often alone, in 30% to 70% of children.[11]

Non-invasive, reliable, accurate surrogate biomarkers of inflammatory activity in children are crucial for disease activity monitoring and assessment of treatment goals. Only 65% of Pediatric gastroenterologists perform repeat endoscopic assessment of disease activity to determine if children achieve mucosal healing in response to treatment as bowel preparation is poorly tolerated, ileal intubation rates are lower than in adults, with as much as 26% of colonoscopies failing to intubate the ileum, and parents may be reluctant to have a child undergo repeat sedation with anesthesia.[12–15] In turn, understanding patient preferences for test accuracy in a non-invasive tight control monitoring is vital to support adherence to a frequent individualized monitoring strategy.[16] Previous monitoring strategies in children relied upon clinical symptoms, yet in the last decade the use of serum and stool biomarkers as surrogate markers for inflammatory activity have proven superior to achieve mucosal healing and prevent disease progression.[17,18] Furthermore, as technology and expertise have advanced, and available serum and stool biomarkers have shown to be imperfect, magnetic resonance enterography, wireless capsule endoscopy, and intestinal ultrasound have emerged, with intestinal ultrasound demonstrating particular promise as a tool for tight control and treat-to-target assessment, acceptable to parents and providers alike to foster adherence and shared understanding for treatment decision making.[19–22]

Unlike adults, clinical trials have left children behind, with only two Federal Drug Administration advanced therapies approved for children with IBD, and pediatric gastroenterologists being forced to fight for off-label use of novel therapies, already approved for years in adults.[23] Thus, optimizing outcomes of limited available therapies by individualizing a precise tight control monitoring strategy with the use of accurate, repeatable, and acceptable non-invasive surrogates is of the most importance in pediatric IBD management today. This review focuses on the journey from old to new, monitoring for the elimination of symptoms as a treatment goal in children to the future of novel non-invasive imaging, serum, and stool biomarkers aimed at disease modification.

CLINICAL SYMPTOM SCORES
Ulcerative colitis

Rates of colectomy in children with ulcerative colitis are as high as 26% and 41% at 5 and 10 years, respectively.[3] In 2007 the Pediatric Ulcerative Colitis Activity Index (PUCAI), a non-invasive clinical score reflecting the previous 2 days of symptoms, was developed and validated using prospective cohorts (Table 1). At its lowest score, a cut-off less than 10 differentiates active from inactive disease with near perfect accuracy (area under the ROC curve 0.99, 95% CI, 0.98–1), and high sensitivity and specificity of 95% and 97%, respectively.[24] Severe baseline PUCAI, more than endoscopic severity, has been shown to be a predictor of colectomy.[4,25–30] Ultimately, the prognosticative utility of the PUCAI at baseline was demonstrated by the Predicting Response to Standardized Pediatric Colitis Therapy (PROTECT) study, a prospective,

Table 1
Pediatric ulcerative colitis and Crohn's disease activity scores

PUCAI (Sum = 0–85)		PCDAI (Sum = 0–110)	
Item	Points	Item	Points
1. Abdominal Pain		*1. Abdominal Pain*	
No pain	0	No pain	0
Pain can be ignored	5	Mild	5
Pain cannot be ignored	10	Moderate/severe	10
2. Rectal bleeding		*2. Stools (per day)*	
None	0	0–1 liquid, no blood	0
Small amount only, < 50% of stools	10	≤ 2 semi-formed w/small blood or 2–5 liquid	5
Small amount with most stools	20	Gross bleeding, or ≥ 6 liquid, or nocturnal diarrhea	10
Large amount (>50% of the stool content)	30	*3. Functioning/General well being*	
3. Stool consistency of most stools		No limitation of activities	0
Formed	0	Occasional difficulty in maintaining age appropriate activities, below par	5
Partially formed	5	Frequent limitation of activity, very poor	10
Completely unformed	10	*4. Hematocrit (%)*	
4. Number of stools per 24 h		< 10 y: > 33, 28–32, < 28	0, 2.5, 5
0–2	0	11–14M: > 35, 30–34, < 30	0, 2.5, 5
3–5	5	15–19M: ≥ 37, 32–36, < 32	0, 2.5, 5
6–8	10	11–19F: ≥34, 29–33, < 29	0, 2.5, 5
>8	15	*5. ESR (mm/h)*	
5. Nocturnal stools (any episode causing wakening)		< 20, 20–50, > 50	0, 2.5, 5
No	0	*6. Albumin (g/dL)*	
Yes	10	≥3.5, 3.1–3.4, ≤ 3.0	0, 5, 10
6. Activity Level		*7. Weight*	
No limitation of activity	0	Weight gain, or voluntary weight stable/loss	0
Occasional limitation of activity	5	Involuntary weight stable, weight loss 1%–9%	5
Severe restricted activity	10	Weight loss ≥ 10%	10

PUCAI (Sum = 0–85)

Disease Activity Cut-Off	AUROC	Sensitivity/Specificity
Severe (>65)	0.91 (0.84–0.98)	79%/85%
Moderate (35–64)	0.91 (0.84–0.98)	79%/85%
Mild (10–34)	0.92 (0.87–0.97)	90%/81%
Inactive (<10)	0.99 (0.98–1)	97%/95%

PCDAI (Sum = 0–110)

8. Height

Diagnosis: <1 channel decrease, >1 but < 2 channel decrease, > 2 channel decrease	0, 5, 10
Follow-up: Velocity > -1SD, < -1SD but >-2SD, < -2SD	0, 5, 10

9. Abdomen

No tenderness, no mass	0
Tenderness, or mass w/out tenderness	5
Tenderness, involuntary guarding, definite mass	10

10. Perirectal disease

None, asymptomatic tags	0
1–2 indolent fistula, scant drainage, no tenderness	5
Active fistula, drainage, tenderness, or abscess	10

11. Extraintestinal manifestations (Fever > 38 > 3 d over past week, definite arthritis, uveitis, E.nodosum)

None, One, > Two	0, 5, 10

Disease Activity Cut-Off

Remission	< 10
Mild	10–30
Moderate-Severe	> 30

29 center inception cohort study of children with newly diagnosed ulcerative colitis undergoing treatment with mesalamine or corticosteroids. A PUCAI score less than 35 predicted week 4 remission (Odds ratio 6.3, 95% CI 3.8–10.4; $P<.0001$) and week 12 corticosteroid-free remission (Odds ratio 2.4, 95% CI 1.4–4.2, $P = .002$), ultimately with PUCAI scores at baseline and 1 month after diagnosis serving as independent predictors of 1-year steroid-free remission.[31,32] PUCAI score at diagnosis and 3 months is also predictive of acute severe ulcerative colitis.[29,33] Day 3 and day 5 PUCAI score of greater than 45 and greater than 70 respectively predict steroid response and the need for additional immunosuppressive therapy.[4,34] Since its creation in 2007 to current day, utilization of a PUCAI score at baseline as a clinical symptom surrogate for disease activity has been and remains an accurate predictor of outcomes and treatment response in children with ulcerative colitis.

Crohn's disease

The Pediatric Crohn's Disease Activity Index (PCDAI) is a non-invasive score combining a 1 week recall of clinical symptoms with physical examination, growth, and laboratory parameters that was developed and validated in 1991.[35] The PCDAI has been the main clinical score for pediatric Crohn's disease drug trials such as the REACH trial for infliximab and IMAgINE trial for adalimumab in which a PCDAI greater than 30 defined active disease at baseline prior to infliximab and adalimumab induction and clinical response for infliximab was PCDAI score decrease $\geq$ 15 and total score $\leq$ 30 at weeks 10, 30, and 54, with clinical remission in this trial defined as a PCDAI $\leq$ 10 and clinical response for adalimumab was a decrease in PCDAI score $\geq$ 15 from baseline at week 4 with a primary endpoint of clinical remission defined as a PCDAI score $\leq$ 10 at week 26.[36,37] However, unlike its clinical symptom score counterpart for pediatric ulcerative colitis, the PUCAI, the PCDAI is cumbersome, requiring laboratory evaluation, physical examination including perirectal examination, and growth assessment. As a result, pediatric gastroenterologists use the PCDAI as a surrogate for inflammatory activity far less often for children with Crohn's disease than the PUCAI for children with ulcerative colitis (48% vs 98%).[38] Additionally, its responsiveness to treatment in a tight control monitoring strategy is not practical. Components of the PCDAI such as growth and weight velocities and physical examination components such as perirectal disease may be longer-term treatment targets. Accordingly, several attempts have been made to modify, shorten, or weight the PCDAI but validation with endoscopy for each remains a continued concern, again limiting its real-world utility in comparison to the PUCAI.[38–42] Recent studies have shown that PCDAI has poor correlation with the simple endoscopic score for Crohn's disease (SES-CD) ($r = 0.33$) and Crohn's disease endoscopic index of severity (CDEIS) ($r = 0.41$) in children at Crohn's disease diagnosis and in response to induction with biologic therapy, $r = .0.34$ and $r = 0.29$ for SES-CD and CDEIS, respectively.[43,44] Additionally, PCDAI at diagnosis was not associated with the need for subsequent treatment.[45,46] Future development of more responsive Crohn's disease patient reported outcomes (PROs) in children will likely be a more accurate reflection of endoscopic activity and more suitable for use as a surrogate marker of Crohn's disease activity during routine clinic visits than the PCDAI and its modified iterations.

C-REACTIVE PROTEIN

C-reactive protein (CRP) is a non-specific, acute phase reactant that rises in response to pro-inflammatory cytokines and as such, is the most commonly used serum biomarker for non-invasive disease activity monitoring in children with IBD, widely available for use in clinics and local laboratories across North America. Additionally, normalization of CRP is an objective treatment target formally recommended in the STRIDE-II guidelines.[10] Yet in a study of 455 children with IBD, CRP was significantly more frequently raised at diagnosis in Crohn's disease than ulcerative colitis (63% vs 22%, P<.0001), leaving many children without a useful non-invasive serum inflammatory biomarker to follow to normalization as a marker of treatment response.[47] When elevated, CRP may serve as an independent predictor of severity and a higher risk of progression to surgery for children with Crohn's disease.[47,48] Elevation in CRP has also not been linked to growth velocity in children with Crohn's disease.[49] In children with newly diagnosed ulcerative colitis, a meta-analysis of four studies found that CRP at diagnosis was not predictive of colectomy.[50] Additionally, CRP has not been associated with disease extension in children diagnosed with limited ulcerative proctitis or left sided-colitis.[51] CRP may be a better predictor of corticosteroid failure in acute severe colitis as an elevated CRP at day 3 and day 5 of intravenous corticosteroid treatment of 99 children admitted for the management of acute severe colitis was shown to be independent predictor (odds ratio = 3.5 (95% CI, 1.4–8.4) of treatment failure.[4]

Additional data on the utility of CRP in adults with Crohn's disease demonstrates added value as a noninvasive biomarker when extrapolated to children. Persistent elevations in CRP in adults with Crohn's disease, in the absence of clinical symptoms, have been associated with hospitalization, poor outcomes, and bowel damage.[52–54] In adults treated with anti-tumor necrosis factor therapy, change in CRP can predict treatment durability, while persistent elevation after 22 weeks can predict a secondary loss of response.[55–57] Lastly, adults with Crohn's disease in clinical remission who attempt to discontinue anti-tumor necrosis factor therapy but have a persistent elevation in CRP, have a 4-fold increased risk of clinical relapse compared to those with a normal CRP.[58,59]

The value of CRP as a non-invasive biomarker begins at diagnosis and/or at treatment initiation. However, for a majority of children with ulcerative colitis, and more than one-third of children with Crohn's disease, CRP has very limited utility, as it is not elevated at diagnosis when there is significant endoscopic activity. Ultimately, in those whom CRP is elevated, combining CRP with other non-invasive markers of inflammation is likely to achieve a more accurate non-invasive assessment of activity for children with IBD.

FECAL CALPROTECTIN

Calprotectin is released from the cytosol of neutrophils, where it is found in abundance, upon activation in the setting of inflammation as it plays a crucial role in the orchestration of the inflammatory response by allowing leukocyte recruitment and transport of arachidonic acid to areas of inflammation.[60] When measured in the stool, calprotectin serves as a non-invasive fecal biomarker accurate for endoscopic activity in children and adults with Crohn's disease and ulcerative colitis. As a diagnostic tool in children presenting with recurrent abdominal pain and/or diarrhea, fecal calprotectin is the most sensitive non-invasive test in children for diagnosing IBD.[61] In a study of 58 children, 26 with Crohn's disease and 32 with ulcerative colitis, fecal calprotectin showed a high correlation with histologic mucosal inflammation (r = 0.655) and was more accurate than clinical symptoms or CRP to detect the presence of active mucosal inflammation on endoscopy with a sensitivity of 94%, specificity of 64%, positive predictive value of 81% and negative predictive value of 87%.[62] In adults with ulcerative colitis, a cut-off fecal calprotectin of less than 192 ug/g was accurate to detect mucosal healing based on both the Mayo Endoscopic Score and Ulcerative Colitis Endoscopic Index of Severity.[63] Similarly, in adults with Crohn's disease, fecal calprotectin correlated more strongly with the SES-CD than CRP or Crohn's Disease Activity Index (CDAI) and a cut-off of 70 ug/g was accurate for the detection of endoscopically active disease with an area under the receiver operating curve of 0.87.[64]

In a multicenter study of children with acute severe colitis, fecal calprotectin was significantly elevated at baseline (4215 (2297–8808) ug/g, but did not perform better than the PUCAI alone at predicting the outcome of treatment with intravenous corticosteroids.[65] For children with IBD, the greatest value for fecal calprotectin may be in its use to predict clinical relapse. In a Canadian study of 40 children (22 Crohn's disease, 18 ulcerative colitis), a cut-off fecal calprotectin of greater than 400 ug/g had an area under the receiver operating curve of 0.83 (95% CI 0.71–0.96 with a sensitivity of 100% and specificity of 75.9%) to predict clinical relapse.[66] Similarly in a study of 104 adults with IBD (49 Crohn's disease, 55 ulcerative colitis), 37 of whom had clinical relapse, a doubling of fecal calprotectin between two consecutive longitudinal collections was associated with a 101% increased risk of relapse (hazard ratio 2.01; 95% CI 1.53–2.65, $P<.001$).[67]

There are several limitations to the use of fecal calprotectin for non-invasive disease activity monitoring, particularly due to the limited, high quality, prospective studies in children. Fecal calprotectin has no ability to discriminate disease extent and location, as a child with inflammation limited to the rectum in ulcerative proctitis may have a higher fecal calprotectin than a children with severe colitis involving the entire colon. Additionally, there is no agreed upon fecal calprotectin cut-off value or percentage decrease for short-term decision making in response to treatment or as a long-term treat-to-target surrogate for mucosal healing. A cut-off value of less than 250 ug/g is generally targeted as a surrogate marker of mucosal healing in adults with IBD, but this has not been studied prospectively in children and remains a critical need in understanding the optimal utilization of fecal calprotectin measurements at various treatment timepoints.[68] Here we propose a fecal calprotectin tight-control monitoring algorithm in children with IBD undergoing treatment with elevated fecal calprotectin at baseline (**Fig. 1**).

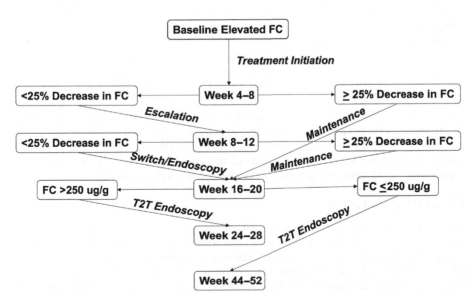

Fig. 1. Fecal calprotectin-based tight control monitoring strategy for children with inflammatory bowel disease to target mucosal healing.

MAGNETIC RESONANCE ENTEROGRAPHY

IBDs are transmural, resulting in inflammation beyond the mucosa to the other four layers of the bowel wall. As such, disease activity monitoring without transmural visualization is incomplete. Incomplete monitoring for transmural disease activity may play a role in creating a barrier to improving outcomes of approved biologic therapies in children. Additionally, ileal non-intubation occurs during 20% to 25% pediatric colonoscopy, requiring another modality to assess disease activity in the ileum even after an invasive procedure.[15]

Magnetic resonance enterography (MRE) is an imaging modality that lacks ionizing radiation but requires oral contrast and in some instances the use of intravenous gadolinium-based contrast agents that is commonly used for transmural disease activity assessment of the ileum in North American children with Crohn's disease. In adults, the Magnetic Resonance Index of Activity (MARIA) tool has become widely accepted as highly accurate for assessing transmural ileal inflammation and has been independently validated with endoscopy.[69] However, the MARIA is cumbersome and takes a long time to calculate, making it impractical for real-time disease activity monitoring. These factors, among others, led to the development of the simplified MARIA (sMARIA) for Crohn's disease in adults. However, the sMARIA is still impractical in children and has rarely been used in pediatric studies, as it requires the use of rectal contrast, which most children and parents are reluctant to undergo.[70]

Recently, the Pediatric Inflammatory Crohn's Magnetic Resonance Enterography Index (PICMI) was developed specifically for pediatric patients with Crohn's disease, becoming the first validated cross-sectional imaging scoring system in children able to discriminate transmural disease activity at a single time point. Additionally, the PICMI was shown to be predictive, with a baseline higher score predictive of disease exacerbation as measured by CRP.[71,72] A PICMI less than 10 was accurate to discriminate between transmural healing and ongoing disease activity. The PICMI is responsive to treatment with agreement between radiologist readers and various MRI machines (interclass correlation coefficient, 0.84, 95% CI 0.79–0.87) and it was a very fast calculation, requiring 2:05 [1:24–2:56] minutes to complete, 80% less time than it takes to calculate the MARIA.

Normalization of bowel wall thickness on MRE has been shown to be an attainable treatment target in children with Crohn's disease initiating treatment with infliximab and azathioprine that correlates strongly with SES-CD on ileocolonoscopy.[73] In a sub-study of the development of the PICMI, 151 children provided a stool sample for calprotectin to match with a complete ileocolonoscopy and concurrent MRE. A fecal calprotectin cut-off of 100 ug/g identified children with deep healing (mucosal and transmural healing) with a 71% sensitivity and 92% specificity.[74] Ultimately, the utilization of the PICMI, combined with fecal calprotectin, may serve as a treatment target for deep healing in children without the need for invasive ileocolonoscopy once additional studies and external validation have been performed.

INTESTINAL ULTRASOUND

Intestinal ultrasound is an emerging non-invasive, real-time, point-of-care, cross-sectional imaging tool that is currently underutilized for disease activity monitoring in both children and adults with Crohn's disease and ulcerative colitis in North America.[75] In Europe, intestinal ultrasound is a central tool in the diagnostic evaluation of pediatric Crohn's disease.[76] Precise monitoring for tight control of IBD activity requires direct visualization, with frequent repetition, with which to make treatment changes based upon. At the current moment, intestinal ultrasound is the only non-invasive tool or biomarker in clinical use with the capability for direct and immediate precision monitoring in children. As a precise monitor of disease activity in children, intestinal ultrasound has several advantages over other modalities and biomarkers mentioned in this review including MRE, CRP, and fecal calprotectin of; (1) no oral contrast, (2) no bowel preparation, (3) real-time results communicated directly to the patient, (4) no sedation or anesthesia, (5) no pain or discomfort, (6) cost-effective, (7) lack of ionizing radiation, and (8) precise assessment of disease location, extent, and severity for both the colon and terminal ileum.[77,78] In children, MRE is not accurate for the evaluation of IBD of the colon. In 140 children with a baseline ileocolonoscopy and MRE within 5 weeks of diagnosis, sMARIA score failed to identify the presence of severe inflammation in all segments of the colon.[79] Additionally, patient centricity is critical to developing a tight control monitoring strategy to enhance adherence. While there is no data to date in children, patients with IBD ranked intestinal ultrasound as their preferred IBD monitoring tool compared to colonoscopy, stool sampling, blood sampling, and additional imaging modalities.[21]

Intestinal Ultrasound versus Magnetic Resonance Enterography

Overall intestinal ultrasound and MRE have similar accuracy for the diagnosis of Crohn's disease complications such as strictures, abscesses, and fistulae.[80] In the largest studies to date, the prospective multi-center METRIC trial including 284 adults, 233 of which had small bowel Crohn's disease, and a multicenter Italian study of 234 adult patients with Crohn's disease, demonstrated that Intestinal ultrasound and MRE are comparable for detection terminal ileal disease. Intestinal ultrasound had a sensitivity and specificity of 92% and 84% while MRE had a sensitivity and specificity of 97% and 96% in the METRIC trial and intestinal ultrasound had a sensitivity and specificity of 96% and 97% in the Italian study compared to 96% and 94% for MRE, respectively.[81,82] MRE was superior to intestinal ultrasound for the detection of small bowel disease extent (80% sensitivity vs 70% sensitivity, respectively). Similarly, in the Italian study, MRE was more accurate than IUS to define small bowel disease extension ($r = 0.69$) and detect fistulae ($\kappa = 0.67$), but comparable for the detection of strictures ($\kappa = 0.82$) and abscesses ($\kappa = 0.88$).

Additional analysis of the METRIC trial debunked a common misconception that intestinal ultrasound is a more operator-dependent imaging modality. Observer agreement for intestinal ultrasound and MRE were similar, with intestinal ultrasound performing better than MRE. Interobserver agreement for MRE was modest for new diagnosis (68% ($\kappa = 0.36$)) and relapsed patients (78% ($\kappa = 0.56$)) and only slight for colonic assessment for new diagnosis (61% ($\kappa = 0.21$)) and relapsed patients (60% ($\kappa = 0.20$)).[83] Interobserver agreement for intestinal ultrasound was higher than MRE in the small bowel for new diagnosis (82% ($\kappa = 0.64$)) and relapsed patients (81% ($\kappa = 0.63$)) and in the colon for new diagnosis (64% ($\kappa = 0.27$)) and relapsed patients (78% ($\kappa = 0.56$)).[84]

Features of Disease Activity on Intestinal Ultrasound in Children

Bowel wall thickness is the most important measure of disease activity on intestinal ultrasound in both children and adults. In adults, a bowel wall thickness cut-off of 3 mm in the terminal ileum is highly accurate to detect endoscopic disease activity with a sensitivity of 88% to 89% and specificity of 93% to 96%.[85,86] Similarly, a BWT cut-off of 3 mm has a sensitivity of 90% and specificity of 96% for endoscopic activity in the colon, with bowel wall thickness showing strong concordance with the Mayo Endoscopic Score in adults with ulcerative colitis.[87,88] In children, especially those between ages 0 to 4 years, there is no consensus definition for normal bowel wall thickness or a cut-off value that correlates with endoscopic activity. A bowel wall thickness less than 1.1 mm is always normal in healthy children and adults, but the upper limit of normal in older healthy children reaches up to 1.9 mm.[89] Multicenter research is needed and currently underway in order to determine normal bowel wall thickness in children of different ages and pubertal status, but a cut-off of 2.5 mm has been proposed as a potentially more accurate cut-off than 3 mm in children for endoscopic activity in the terminal ileum and colon, but this needs to be proven and validated.[77]

In order to differentiate children with inflammation from those without who have a bowel wall thickness less than 3 mm, and to help understand the components of active versus chronic inflammation present, assessment of bowel wall hyperemia by color Doppler signal should be performed as part of the standard disease activity assessment. To date, there has been no validated quantification tool for hyperemia, such as the Limberg score used in adults, in children. However, the only two pediatric intestinal ultrasound scores developed and validated with endoscopy both found the presence of hyperemia to be independent predictors of endoscopic activity, further emphasizing the importance of color Doppler assessment in the standardized exam of the bowel in children with IBD.[90,91]

Pediatric Intestinal Ultrasound Activity Scores

To date, there are 2 specific intestinal ultrasound scores that have been developed for children with IBD. In a study of 50 children with ulcerative colitis and suspected disease flare up, intestinal ultrasound and colonoscopy were performed with intestinal ultrasound demonstrating a 90% (95% CI 0.82–0.96) concordance with endoscopic activity in the colon.[90] Intestinal ultrasound measures of bowel wall thickness, increased vascularity on color Doppler signal, absence of normal haustration and stratification were all independently predictive of endoscopic severity and the Civitelli ulcerative colitis index consists of these 5 parameters (**Table 2**). A score greater than 2 had a sensitivity of 100% and specificity of 93% (area under the ROC = 0 .98). The second score, the Simple Pediatric Activity Ultrasound Score (SPAUSS) was developed in 75 children with IBD (56 Crohn's disease, 15 ulcerative colitis, and 4 inflammatory bowel disease unclassified).[91] Intestinal ultrasound was highly accurate to detect endoscopic disease activity, 100% sensitive and specific (area under the ROC = 1.00 to detect ileal disease and 86.6% sensitive and 100% specific to detect colonic disease (area under the ROC = 0.92). The SPAUSS consists of only 3 intestinal ultrasound parameters, bowel wall thickness, hyperemia on color Doppler signal, and inflammatory fat. A score greater than 7 was the most sensitive and specific for predicting active disease with an area under the ROC = 0.82 (95% CI 0.72–0.92). External validation with objective endoscopic scores and assessment of treatment responsiveness is needed for both scores to understand how to better use them and identify target score changes at different treatment intervals. Once that occurs, it is likely that changes in intestinal ultrasound scores will be able to serve as early targets in the treatment course of children with IBD, allowing to providers to confidently make treatment decisions with a direct, non-invasive surrogate of endoscopic activity without the need for actual endoscopy requiring bowel preparation and sedation with anesthesia.

Monitoring treatment response on intestinal ultrasound

While there are multiple studies assessing treatment responsiveness of intestinal ultrasound in adults with IBD, there are only two to date in children. The first study of 28 children with newly diagnosed ileal Crohn's disease initiating treatment with infliximab

Table 2
Pediatric intestinal ultrasound scores

Score	Bowel Wall Thickness	Bowel Wall Hyperemia	Loss of Bowel Wall Stratification	Abnormal Haustrations	Inflammatory Fat
Civitelli UC Index (0–4)	0: ≤ 3 mm 1: > 3 mm	0: Absent 1: Present	0: No loss 1: Loss	0: Normal 1: Abnormal	
SPAUSS (1–14)	1: ≤ 3.9 mm 4: 4–6.9 mm 6: ≥ 7 mm	0: Absent 1: Mild activity 2: Moderate/Severe activity			0: Absent 1: Mild 6: Moderate/Severe

was conducted in which intestinal ultrasound was performed at approximately 2 weeks, 1 month, 3 months, and 6 months after initiation. By 2 weeks after treatment initiation, there was a decrease in the mean bowel wall thickness from 5.6 ± 1.8 mm to 4.7 ± 1.7 mm ($P = .02$), length of bowel segment involved from 12.0 ± 5.4 cm to 9.1 ± 5.3 cm ($P = .02$), and hyperemia on color Doppler signal ($P = .005$).[92] Through 6 months, linear mixed models confirmed that bowel wall thickness, length of disease involvement and bowel wall hyperemia on color Doppler signal continue to improve over time. Similarly, in a small pilot study from our center of 13 children with ileal Crohn's disease initiating treatment with infliximab, bowel wall hyperemia and bowel wall segment length involved decreased significantly after induction with fecal calprotectin moderately correlating with a decrease in the bowel segment length post-induction ($r = 0.57$, $P = .04$).[93]

Targeting reduction in bowel wall thickness and hyperemia on intestinal ultrasound early and repeatedly after the initiation of treatment in children with inflammatory bowel disease is likely to serve as novel, non-invasive, targets in the near future as current research is ongoing. Transmural healing (normalization of bowel wall thickness and hyperemia) is not formally recommended as a treatment target in the STRIDE-II guidelines, but may be an attainable target, even as early as post-induction, for children who with newly diagnosed IBD initiating effective treatments (**Fig. 2**).

WIRELESS CAPSULE ENDOSCOPY

Up to 30% of children with Crohn's disease will have isolated ileal or small bowel Crohn's disease which presents a unique challenge for monitoring disease activity and assessing for healing, especially with higher ileal non-intubation rates in pediatric colonoscopy than adults.[11,15] In older children and adolescents who can swallow large pills without requiring endoscopic placement, wireless capsule endoscopy is a practical non-invasive modality to monitor for mucosal healing in a treat-to-target approach for children with small bowel Crohn's disease. In a prospective study of children with small bowel Crohn's disease undergoing wireless capsule endoscopy

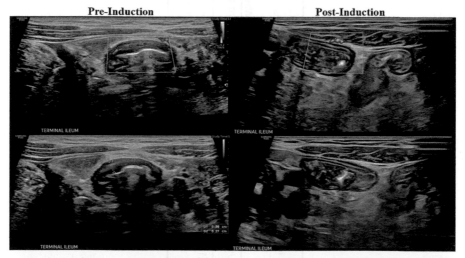

Fig. 2. Post-induction normalization of bowel wall thickness and hyperemia on intestinal ultrasound. Transmural healing as represented by normalization of the terminal ileum post-induction after 4 weeks of adalimumab therapy in a child with newly diagnosed ileal Crohn's disease.

to assess mucosal healing at baseline, week 24, and week 52 in a treat-to-target approach, findings on wireless capsule endoscopy led to a change in therapy for 74% of children at baseline and 23% of children at 24 weeks. Using a treat-to-target approach for mucosal healing on wireless capsule endoscopy yielded an increase in the proportion of children with mucosal healing and deep remission from 21% at baseline to 54% at week 24% and 58% at week 52 with only 4% of patients having non-response to treatment.[19]

SUMMARY

Traditional monitoring strategies for children with IBD have relied upon monitoring clinical symptoms and serum inflammatory markers. However, this monitoring strategy offers an incomplete evaluation of disease activity and a strategy that has resulted in the stagnation of clinical outcomes from available advanced therapies for children for quite some time. Without novel therapies readily available and approved by the Federal Drug Administration, pediatric gastroenterologists need to switch gears and adopt novel tight control monitoring strategies within the treat-to-target framework to maximize the therapies available today.

In order to achieve this, patient centric, accurate, real-time non-invasive surrogates of IBD activity in the small intestine and colon are needed. Intestinal ultrasound represents an ideal emerging tool for this purpose, with more training needed to develop expertise and multicenter studies in children to optimize its use for tight control and treatment decision making. Concurrently, utilizing a combination of clinical symptom scores, CRP, fecal calprotectin, changes on intestinal ultrasound, the PICMI on MRE, and wireless capsule endoscopy in a precision strategy based on a patients baseline IBD location and behavior will emerge in the near future and it is likely that research will show that this precision approach leads to deep healing and disease modification, thus altering the natural history of pediatric IBD while simultaneously reducing the need for repeated intolerable procedures.

CLINICS CARE POINTS

- Only two biologic therapies are approved for the treatment of children with inflammatory bowel disease, as clinical symptoms alone are unreliable to detect inflammation, non-invasive, tight control monitoring strategies are needed to achieve and maintain endoscopic remission.

- When monitoring clinical symptoms and their response to treatment, use of the PUCAI in children with ulcerative colitis, can be an accurate non-invasive surrogate for endoscopic inflammation and predictive of outcomes.

- CRP, the most common serum biomarker, is more commonly elevated in children with Crohn's disease than ulcerative colitis, however for many it is not elevated at baseline, often leaving children without a serum biomarker to follow treatment response.

- Fecal calprotectin is an accurate, non-invasive stool biomarker of disease activity, particularly in ulcerative colitis, with the strongest evidence for its ability to predict clinical relapse in children with ulcerative colitis in clinical remission.

- The PICMI is the first pediatric Crohn's disease MRE index that is easily and quickly calculated, now validated to discriminate transmural disease activity at a single point and responsive to treatment.

- Intestinal ultrasound has emerged as an ideal, non-invasive, point-of-care disease activity monitoring tool in children with both Crohn's disease and ulcerative colitis.

• Intestinal ultrasound is accurate to detect endoscopic disease activity in children with IBD and capable of monitoring treatment response, particularly early in the course.

FUNDING

Intestinal Ultrasound research at Mount Sinai is supported by Henry and Elaine Kaufman.

DISCLOSURE

M.T. Dolinger is a consultant for Neurologica corp., a subsidiary of Samsung Electronics Co., ltd.

REFERENCES

1. Torres J, Mehandru S, Colombel JF, et al. Crohn's disease. Lancet 2017; 389(10080):1741–55.
2. Krugliak Cleveland N, Torres J, Rubin DT. What Does Disease Progression Look Like in Ulcerative Colitis, and How Might It Be Prevented? Gastroenterology 2022; 162(5):1396–408.
3. Van Limbergen J, Russell RK, Drummond HE, et al. Definition of Phenotypic Characteristics of Childhood-Onset Inflammatory Bowel Disease. Gastroenterology 2008;135(4):1114–22.
4. Turner D, Walsh CM, Benchimol EI, et al. Severe paediatric ulcerative colitis: incidence, outcomes and optimal timing for second-line therapy. Gut 2008;57(3): 331–8.
5. Benchimol EI, Bernstein CN, Bitton A, et al. Trends in Epidemiology of Pediatric Inflammatory Bowel Disease in Canada: Distributed Network Analysis of Multiple Population-Based Provincial Health Administrative Databases. Am J Gastroenterol 2017;112(7):1120–34.
6. Vernier–Massouille G, Balde M, Salleron J, et al. Natural History of Pediatric Crohn's Disease: A Population-Based Cohort Study. Gastroenterology 2008; 135(4):1106–13.
7. Chouraki V, Savoye G, Dauchet L, et al. The changing pattern of Crohn's disease incidence in northern France: a continuing increase in the 10- to 19-year-old age bracket (1988-2007): Epidemiology of inflammatory bowel disease. Aliment Pharmacol Ther 2011;33(10):1133–42.
8. Ye Y, Manne S, Treem WR, et al. Prevalence of Inflammatory Bowel Disease in Pediatric and Adult Populations: Recent Estimates From Large National Databases in the United States, 2007–2016. Inflamm Bowel Dis 2019. https://doi.org/10. 1093/ibd/izz182. izz182.
9. Colombel JF, D'haens G, Lee WJ, et al. Outcomes and Strategies to Support a Treat-to-target Approach in Inflammatory Bowel Disease: A Systematic Review. J Crohns Colitis 2020;14(2):254–66.
10. Turner D, Ricciuto A, Lewis A, et al. STRIDE-II: An Update on the Selecting Therapeutic Targets in Inflammatory Bowel Disease (STRIDE) Initiative of the International Organization for the Study of IBD (IOIBD): Determining Therapeutic Goals for Treat-to-Target strategies in IBD. Gastroenterology 2021;160(5):1570–83.
11. Cuffari C, Dubinsky M, Darbari A, et al. Crohn's Jejunoileitis: The Pediatrician's Perspective on Diagnosis and Management. Inflamm Bowel Dis 2005;11(7): 696–704.

12. Moses J, Sandberg K, Winberry G, et al. Clinical Practice Survey of Repeat Endoscopy in Pediatric Inflammatory Bowel Disease in North America. J Pediatr Gastroenterol Nutr 2021;73(1):61–6.
13. Hochman JA, Figueroa J, Duner E, et al. Diagnostic Yield Variation with Colonoscopy among Pediatric Endoscopists. Dig Dis 2020;38(5):421–30.
14. Pasquarella CS, Kaplan B, Mahajan L, et al. A Single-center Review of Pediatric Colonoscopy Quality Indicators. J Pediatr Gastroenterol Nutr 2019;68(5):648–54.
15. de Bie CI, Buderus S, Sandhu BK, et al. Diagnostic Workup of Paediatric Patients With Inflammatory Bowel Disease in Europe: Results of a 5-Year Audit of the EUROKIDS Registry. J Pediatr Gastroenterol Nutr 2012;54(3):374–80.
16. Barsky M, Meserve J, Le H, et al. Understanding Determinants of Patient Preferences Between Stool Tests and Colonoscopy for the Assessment of Disease Activity in Inflammatory Bowel Disease. Dig Dis Sci 2021;66(8):2564–9.
17. Colombel JF, Panaccione R, Bossuyt P, et al. Effect of tight control management on Crohn's disease (CALM): a multicentre, randomised, controlled phase 3 trial. Lancet 2017;390(10114):2779–89.
18. Ungaro RC, Yzet C, Bossuyt P, et al. Deep Remission at 1 Year Prevents Progression of Early Crohn's Disease. Gastroenterology 2020;159(1):139–47.
19. Oliva S, Aloi M, Viola F, et al. A Treat to Target Strategy Using Panenteric Capsule Endoscopy in Pediatric Patients With Crohn's Disease. Clin Gastroenterol Hepatol 2019;17(10):2060–7.e1.
20. Christensen KR, Steenholdt C, Buhl S, et al. A systematic monitoring approach to biologic therapies in inflammatory bowel disease: patients' and physicians' preferences and adherence. Scand J Gastroenterol 2022;57(3):274–81.
21. Rajagopalan A, Sathananthan D, An Y, et al. Gastrointestinal ultrasound in inflammatory bowel disease care: Patient perceptions and impact on disease-related knowledge. JGH Open 2020;4(2):267–72.
22. Friedman AB, Asthana A, Knowles SR, et al. Effect of point-of-care gastrointestinal ultrasound on decision-making and management in inflammatory bowel disease. Aliment Pharmacol Ther 2021;54(5):652–66.
23. Turner D, Griffiths AM, Wilson D, et al. Designing clinical trials in paediatric inflammatory bowel diseases: a PIBDnet commentary. Gut 2020;69(1):32–41.
24. Turner D, Otley AR, Mack D, et al. Development, Validation, and Evaluation of a Pediatric Ulcerative Colitis Activity Index: A Prospective Multicenter Study. Gastroenterology 2007;133(2):423–32.
25. Falcone R. Predicting the need for colectomy in pediatric patients with ulcerative colitis. J Gastrointest Surg 2000;4(2):201–6.
26. Malaty H, Abraham BP, Mehta S, et al. The natural history of ulcerative colitis in a pediatric population: a follow-up population- based cohort study. Clin Exp Gastroenterol 2013;77. https://doi.org/10.2147/CEG.S40259.
27. Hochart A, Gower-Rousseau C, Sarter H, et al. Ulcerative proctitis is a frequent location of paediatric-onset UC and not a minor disease: a population-based study. Gut 2017;66(11):1912–7.
28. Kelley-Quon LI, Jen HC, Ziring DA, et al. Predictors of Proctocolectomy in Children With Ulcerative Colitis. J Pediatr Gastroenterol Nutr 2012;55(5):534–40.
29. Nambu R, ichiro HS, Kubota M, et al. Difference between early onset and late-onset pediatric ulcerative colitis: Early onset colitis phenotype. Pediatr Int 2016; 58(9):862–6.
30. Hyams JS, Brimacombe M, Haberman Y, et al. Clinical and Host Biological Factors Predict Colectomy Risk in Children Newly Diagnosed With Ulcerative Colitis. Inflamm Bowel Dis 2022;28(2):151–60.

31. Hyams JS, Davis S, Mack DR, et al. Factors associated with early outcomes following standardised therapy in children with ulcerative colitis (PROTECT): a multicentre inception cohort study. Lancet Gastroenterol Hepatol 2017;2(12): 855–68.

32. Hyams JS, Davis Thomas S, Gotman N, et al. Clinical and biological predictors of response to standardised paediatric colitis therapy (PROTECT): a multicentre inception cohort study. Lancet 2019;393(10182):1708–20.

33. Barabino A, egaldo L, Castellano E, et al. Severe attack of ulcerative colitis in children: retrospective clinical survey. Dig Liver Dis 2002;34(1):44–9.

34. Turner D, Mack D, Leleiko N, et al. Severe Pediatric Ulcerative Colitis: A Prospective Multicenter Study of Outcomes and Predictors of Response. Gastroenterology 2010;138(7):2282–91.

35. Hyams JS, Ferry GD, Mandel FS, et al. Development and Validation of a Pediatric Crohn's Disease Activity Index. J Pediatr Gastroenterol Nutr 1991;12(4):439–47.

36. Hyams J, Crandall W, Kugathasan S, et al. Induction and Maintenance Infliximab Therapy for the Treatment of Moderate-to-Severe Crohn's Disease in Children. Gastroenterology 2007;132(3):863–73.

37. Hyams JS, Griffiths A, Markowitz J, et al. Safety and Efficacy of Adalimumab for Moderate to Severe Crohn's Disease in Children. Gastroenterology 2012;143(2): 365–74.e2.

38. Kappelman MD, Crandall WV, Colletti RB, et al. Short pediatric Crohn's disease activity index for quality improvement and observational research. Inflamm Bowel Dis 2011;17(1):112–7.

39. Turner D, Griffiths AM, Walters TD, et al. Mathematical weighting of the pediatric Crohn's disease activity index (PCDAI) and comparison with its other short versions. Inflamm Bowel Dis 2012;18(1):55–62.

40. Turner D, Levine A, Walters TD, et al. Which PCDAI Version Best Reflects Intestinal Inflammation in Pediatric Crohn Disease? J Pediatr Gastroenterol Nutr 2017;64(2):254–60.

41. Shepanski MA, Markowitz JE, Mamula P, et al. Is an Abbreviated Pediatric Crohn's Disease Activity Index Better Than the Original? J Pediatr Gastroenterol Nutr 2004;39(1):68–72.

42. Loonen HJ, Griffiths AM, Merkus MP, et al. A Critical Assessment of Items on the Pediatric Crohn's Disease Activity Index. J Pediatr Gastroenterol Nutr 2003; 36(1):90–5.

43. Zubin G, Peter L. Predicting Endoscopic Crohn's Disease Activity Before and After Induction Therapy in Children: A Comprehensive Assessment of PCDAI, CRP, and Fecal Calprotectin. Inflamm Bowel Dis 2015;1. https://doi.org/10.1097/MIB. 0000000000000388.

44. Yu Y, Zhao H, Luo Y, et al. Poor Concordance Between Clinical Activity and Endoscopic Severity in Pediatric Crohn's Disease: Before and After Induction Therapy. Dig Dis Sci 2022;67(3):997–1006.

45. Jacobstein DA, Mamula P, Markowitz JE, et al. Predictors of Immunomodulator Use as Early Therapy in Pediatric Crohn's Disease. J Clin Gastroenterol 2006; 40(2):145–8.

46. Olbjørn C, Nakstad B, Småstuen MC, et al. Early anti-TNF treatment in pediatric Crohn's disease. Predictors of clinical outcome in a population-based cohort of newly diagnosed patients. Scand J Gastroenterol 2014;49(12):1425–31.

47. Henderson P, Kennedy NA, Van Limbergen JE, et al. Serum C-reactive Protein and CRP Genotype in Pediatric Inflammatory Bowel Disease: Influence on

Phenotype, Natural History, and Response to Therapy. Inflamm Bowel Dis 2015; 21(3):596–605.

48. De Greef E, Mahachie John JM, Hoffman I, et al. Profile of pediatric Crohn's disease in Belgium. J Crohns Colitis 2013;7(11):e588–98.

49. Sawczenko A, Ballinger AB, Savage MO, et al. Clinical Features Affecting Final Adult Height in Patients With Pediatric-Onset Crohn's Disease. Pediatrics 2006; 118(1):124–9.

50. Orlanski-Meyer E, Aardoom M, Ricciuto A, et al. Predicting Outcomes in Pediatric Ulcerative Colitis for Management Optimization: Systematic Review and Consensus Statements From the Pediatric Inflammatory Bowel Disease–Ahead Program. Gastroenterology 2021;160(1):378–402.e22.

51. Aloi M, D'Arcangelo G, Pofi F, et al. Presenting features and disease course of pediatric ulcerative colitis. J Crohns Colitis 2013;7(11):e509–15.

52. Bhattacharya A, Rao BB, Koutroubakis IE, et al. Silent Crohn's Disease Predicts Increased Bowel Damage During Multiyear Follow-up: The Consequences of Under-reporting Active Inflammation. Inflamm Bowel Dis 2016;22(11):2665–71.

53. Click B, Vargas EJ, Anderson AM, et al. Silent Crohn's Disease: Asymptomatic Patients with Elevated C-reactive Protein Are at Risk for Subsequent Hospitalization. Inflamm Bowel Dis 2015;1. https://doi.org/10.1097/MIB.0000000000000516.

54. Oh K, Oh EH, Baek S, et al. Elevated C-reactive protein level during clinical remission can predict poor outcomes in patients with Crohn's disease. PLoS One 2017; 12(6):e0179266.

55. Reinisch W, Wang Y, Oddens BJ, et al. C-reactive protein, an indicator for maintained response or remission to infliximab in patients with Crohn's disease: a post-hoc analysis from ACCENT I. Aliment Pharmacol Ther 2012;35(5):568–76.

56. Cornillie F, Hanauer SB, Diamond RH, et al. Postinduction serum infliximab trough level and decrease of C-reactive protein level are associated with durable sustained response to infliximab: a retrospective analysis of the ACCENT I trial. Gut 2014; 63(11):1721–7.

57. Echarri A, Ollero V, Barreiro-de Acosta M, et al. Clinical, biological, and endoscopic responses to adalimumab in antitumor necrosis factor-naive Crohn's disease: predictors of efficacy in clinical practice. Eur J Gastroenterol Hepatol 2015; 27(4):430–5.

58. Louis E, Mary J, Vernier–Massouille G, et al. Maintenance of Remission Among Patients With Crohn's Disease on Antimetabolite Therapy After Infliximab Therapy Is Stopped. Gastroenterology 2012;142(1):63–70.e5.

59. Roblin X, Marotte H, Leclerc M, et al. Combination of C-reactive Protein, Infliximab Trough Levels, and Stable but Not Transient Antibodies to Infliximab Are Associated With Loss of Response to Infliximab in Inflammatory Bowel Disease. J Crohns Colitis 2015;9(7):525–31.

60. Jukic A, Bakiri L, Wagner EF, et al. Calprotectin: from biomarker to biological function. Gut 2021;70(10):1978–88.

61. Dilillo D, Zuccotti GV, Galli E, et al. Noninvasive testing in the management of children with suspected inflammatory bowel disease. Scand J Gastroenterol 2019; 54(5):586–91.

62. Berni Canani R, Terrin G, Rapacciuolo L, et al. Faecal calprotectin as reliable noninvasive marker to assess the severity of mucosal inflammation in children with inflammatory bowel disease. Dig Liver Dis 2008;40(7):547–53.

63. Theede K, Holck S, Ibsen P, et al. Level of Fecal Calprotectin Correlates With Endoscopic and Histologic Inflammation and Identifies Patients With Mucosal Healing in Ulcerative Colitis. Clin Gastroenterol Hepatol 2015;13(11):1929–36.e1.

64. Schoepfer AM, Beglinger C, Straumann A, et al. Fecal Calprotectin Correlates More Closely With the Simple Endoscopic Score for Crohn's Disease (SES-CD) than CRP, Blood Leukocytes, and the CDAI. Am J Gastroenterol 2010;105(1): 162–9.

65. Turner D, Leach ST, Mack D, et al. Faecal calprotectin, lactoferrin, M2-pyruvate kinase and S100A12 in severe ulcerative colitis: a prospective multicentre comparison of predicting outcomes and monitoring response. Gut 2010;59(9): 1207–12.

66. Kittanakom S, Shajib MdS, Garvie K, et al. Comparison of Fecal Calprotectin Methods for Predicting Relapse of Pediatric Inflammatory Bowel Disease. Can J Gastroenterol Hepatol 2017;2017:1–10.

67. Zhulina Y, Cao Y, Amcoff K, et al. The prognostic significance of faecal calprotectin in patients with inactive inflammatory bowel disease. Aliment Pharmacol Ther 2016;44(5):495–504.

68. Lin JF, Chen JM, Zuo JH, et al. Meta-analysis: Fecal Calprotectin for Assessment of Inflammatory Bowel Disease Activity. Inflamm Bowel Dis 2014;20(8):1407–15.

69. Rimola J, Rodriguez S, Garcia-Bosch O, et al. Magnetic resonance for assessment of disease activity and severity in ileocolonic Crohn's disease. Gut 2009; 58(8):1113–20.

70. Ordás I, Rimola J, Alfaro I, et al. Development and Validation of a Simplified Magnetic Resonance Index of Activity for Crohn's Disease. Gastroenterology 2019; 157(2):432–9.e1.

71. Focht G, Cytter-Kuint R, Greer MLC, et al. Development, Validation, and Evaluation of the Pediatric Inflammatory Crohn's Magnetic Resonance Enterography Index From the ImageKids Study. Gastroenterology 2022;163(5):1306–20.

72. Dolinger MT, Dubinsky MC. The Pediatric Inflammatory Crohn's Magnetic Resonance Enterography Index: A Step Forward for Transmural Pediatric Crohn's Disease Monitoring and Healing. Gastroenterology 2022;163(5):1166–7.

73. Kang B, Choi SY, Chi S, et al. Baseline Wall Thickness Is Lower in Mucosa-Healed Segments 1 Year After Infliximab in Pediatric Crohn Disease Patients. J Pediatr Gastroenterol Nutr 2017;64(2):279–85.

74. Weinstein-Nakar I, Focht G, Church P, et al. Associations Among Mucosal and Transmural Healing and Fecal Level of Calprotectin in Children With Crohn's Disease. Clin Gastroenterol Hepatol 2018;16(7):1089–97.e4.

75. Bryant RV, Friedman AB, Wright EK, et al. Gastrointestinal ultrasound in inflammatory bowel disease: an underused resource with potential paradigm-changing application. Gut 2018;67(5):973–85.

76. van Rheenen PF, Aloi M, Assa A, et al. The Medical Management of Paediatric Crohn's Disease: an ECCO-ESPGHAN Guideline Update. J Crohns Colitis 2021;15(2):171–94.

77. Kellar A, Dolinger M, Novak KL, et al. Intestinal Ultrasound for the Pediatric Gastroenterologist: A Guide for Inflammatory Bowel Disease Monitoring in Children. J Pediatr Gastroenterol Nutr 2022. https://doi.org/10.1097/MPG.00000000 00003649.

78. Wilkens R, Dolinger M, Burisch J, et al. Point-of-Care Testing and Home Testing: Pragmatic Considerations for Widespread Incorporation of Stool Tests, Serum Tests, and Intestinal Ultrasound. Gastroenterology 2022;162(5):1476–92.

79. Lepus CA, Moote DJ, Bao S, et al. Simplified Magnetic Resonance Index of Activity Is Useful for Terminal Ileal but not Colonic Disease in Pediatric Crohn Disease. J Pediatr Gastroenterol Nutr 2022;74(5):610–6.

80. Panés J, Bouzas R, Chaparro M, et al. Systematic review: the use of ultrasonography, computed tomography and magnetic resonance imaging for the diagnosis, assessment of activity and abdominal complications of Crohn's disease: Systematic review: cross-sectional imaging in Crohn's disease. Aliment Pharmacol Ther 2011;34(2):125–45.

81. Taylor SA, Mallett S, Bhatnagar G, et al. Diagnostic accuracy of magnetic resonance enterography and small bowel ultrasound for the extent and activity of newly diagnosed and relapsed Crohn's disease (METRIC): a multicentre trial. Lancet Gastroenterol Hepatol 2018;3(8):548–58.

82. Castiglione F, Mainenti PP, De Palma GD, et al. Noninvasive Diagnosis of Small Bowel Crohn's Disease: Direct Comparison of Bowel Sonography and Magnetic Resonance Enterography. Inflamm Bowel Dis 2013;19(5):991–8.

83. Bhatnagar G, Mallett S, Quinn L, et al. Interobserver variation in the interpretation of magnetic resonance enterography in Crohn's disease. Br J Radiol 2022; 95(1134):20210995.

84. METRIC study investigators, Bhatnagar G, Quinn L, et al. Observer agreement for small bowel ultrasound in Crohn's disease: results from the METRIC trial. Abdom Radiol 2020;45(10):3036–45.

85. Dong J, Wang H, Zhao J, et al. Ultrasound as a diagnostic tool in detecting active Crohn's disease: a meta-analysis of prospective studies. Eur Radiol 2014;24(1): 26–33.

86. Fraquelli M, Colli A, Casazza G, et al. Role of US in Detection of Crohn Disease: Meta-Analysis. Radiology 2005;236(1):95–101.

87. Horsthuis K, Bipat S, Bennink RJ, et al. Inflammatory Bowel Disease Diagnosed with US, MR, Scintigraphy, and CT: Meta-analysis of Prospective Studies. Radiology 2008;247(1):64–79.

88. Antonelli E, Giuliano V, Casella G, et al. Ultrasonographic assessment of colonic wall in moderate–severe ulcerative colitis: Comparison with endoscopic findings. Dig Liver Dis 2011;43(9):703–6.

89. van Wassenaer EA, de Voogd FAE, van Rijn RR, et al. Bowel ultrasound measurements in healthy children — systematic review and meta-analysis. Pediatr Radiol 2020;50(4):501–8.

90. Civitelli F, Di Nardo G, Oliva S, et al. Ultrasonography of the Colon in Pediatric Ulcerative Colitis: A Prospective, Blind, Comparative Study with Colonoscopy. J Pediatr 2014;165(1):78–84.e2.

91. Kellar A, Wilson S, Kaplan G, et al. The Simple Pediatric Activity Ultrasound Score (SPAUSS) for the Accurate Detection of Pediatric Inflammatory Bowel Disease. J Pediatr Gastroenterol Nutr 2019;69(1):e1–6.

92. Dillman JR, Dehkordy SF, Smith EA, et al. Defining the ultrasound longitudinal natural history of newly diagnosed pediatric small bowel Crohn disease treated with infliximab and infliximab–azathioprine combination therapy. Pediatr Radiol 2017; 47(8):924–34.

93. Dolinger MT, Choi JJ, Phan BL, et al. Use of Small Bowel Ultrasound to Predict Response to Infliximab Induction in Pediatric Crohn's Disease. J Clin Gastroenterol 2021;55(5):429–32.

Choosing the Right Therapy at the Right Time for Pediatric Inflammatory Bowel Disease: Does Sequence Matter

Elizabeth A. Spencer, MD, MSc

KEYWORDS

- Pediatric • IBD • Crohn's disease • Ulcerative colitis • Early effective therapy
- Precision medicine • Biologic therapies

KEY POINTS

- Despite the enlarging therapeutic armamentarium in inflammatory bowel disease (IBD), it is still plagued by a therapeutic ceiling that precision medicine may overcome.
- The benefits of early effective therapy are clear in CD but not UC. Pediatric data is lacking in either subtype.
- Clinical characteristics, traditional laboratory values, and pharmacogenomics can all be used to understand patient prognosis to inform treatment choice.
- There are increasing head-to-head trials allowing a better understanding of the importance of therapeutic sequence.
- Therapeutic choice requires a holistic approach, examining a patient's phenotype, severity, and numerous other clinical factors in addition to weighing a patient's personal choices and cost considerations.

INTRODUCTION

Despite the enlarging therapeutic armamentarium in inflammatory bowel disease (IBD), it is still plagued by a therapeutic ceiling, with response to therapy in clinical trials typically not exceeding 30% of patients.[1] Furthermore, those who ultimately find the correct therapy often do so only after failing multiple trials of medications, which can be disabling, psychologically stressful, and with permanent consequences for the bowel wall. A comprehensive solution to this problem can be attained through precision medicine to allow for the selection of all the "rights" – the right patient, right therapy, right time, right dose, and right monitoring strategy[2]; Alexander Nasr and Phillip Minar's article, "The Role of Therapeutic Drug Monitoring in Children"; and Michael

Division of Pediatric Gastroenterology & Nutrition, Department of Pediatrics, Icahn School of Medicine, Mount Sinai, 17 East 102nd Street, 5th Floor, New York, NY 10029, USA
E-mail address: Elizabeth.spencer@mssm.edu

Gastroenterol Clin N Am 52 (2023) 517–534
https://doi.org/10.1016/j.gtc.2023.05.006
0889-8553/23/© 2023 Elsevier Inc. All rights reserved.

Todd Dolinger's article, "The Role of Noninvasive Surrogates of Inflammation in Monitoring Pediatric IBD: The Old and the New," in this issue have discussed two such tactics that are currently available of choosing the correct dose and implementing the correct monitoring strategy to verify response, respectively. This review will discuss the critical process of pairing the right patient with right therapy at the right time, which are all interrelated. Given that much of the data on this topic comes from adult populations, adult and pediatric data will both be presented. We will first focus on the shift to early effective therapy, where gastroenterologists strive to position therapies that are more likely to be effective as early as possible in the treatment course, and its benefits over the historical practice of stepping up through ineffective therapies with the attendant, unnecessary accrual of bowel wall damage. We will then discuss promising future strategies of patient profiling to better sift through heterogenous patients with IBD to identify patients at high risk for complication as well as the underlying biological pathways underpinning their disease. Finally, we will discuss the practical considerations that drive treatment selection, particularly the impact of the therapeutic sequence.

THE RIGHT TIME: EARLY EFFECTIVE THERAPY
Treating a Progressive Disease

IBD, which includes Crohn's disease (CD)[3] and ulcerative colitis (UC),[4] is a heterogenous chronic disease that is progressive in nature with associated irreversible bowel wall injury. Unfortunately, all current treatments are geared toward extinguishing inflammation, but there are no therapies for reversing the damage to the bowel wall. As such, the natural history of the disease leads to complication(s) that medicines cannot reverse, often resulting in surgery.[5] Initiating therapy before the accrual of this untreatable damage has increasingly been recognized as a critical pathway to change the natural history of the disease.

In CD, fibrosis is a well-known complication, leading to strictures that will affect one-third of patients at some point in their disease course.[3] This may be even more relevant in patients with pediatric IBD. Pediatric-onset CD has been shown to have a more severe phenotype than adult-onset CD,[6] leading to the suggestion that pediatric patients with CD may benefit even more from early, more-aggressive therapy to prevent the resultant damage from chronic, uncontrolled inflammation over an inherently prolonged disease duration.[7]

UC has only more recently being recognized as a progressive disease. Over half of patients with UC will have disease extension, and colonic fibrotic strictures can be seen in a small proportion of patients. Additionally, disease duration, severity, and activity have been associated with increasing colorectal cancer risk.[8]

Hindered by History: Step-Up Therapy

Historically, IBD was treated with "step-up" therapy. This was the convention of requiring failure of less effective medications, like mesalamine and thiopurines, before starting biologics in all patients with IBD, including those with moderate-to-severe disease. Yet, there is increasing evidence that tactics such as this cause patients to miss an important "window of opportunity" to permanently alter their disease course by quickly and durably snuffing the fires of inflammation, eradicating bowel wall damage and the resultant complications.[9] This has led to a change in conventions from "step-up" to "early effective" therapy; early effective therapy is the tactic of pairing the initial treatment modality with the severity and phenotype of the disease, often leading to the upfront usage of biologic therapies (**Fig. 1**).

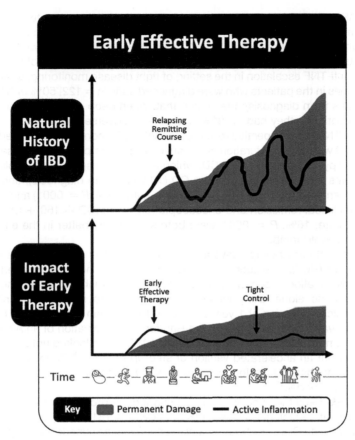

Fig. 1. Comparison of bowel wall damage and active inflammation over time in Untreated IBD and IBD treated early with effective therapy.

While this is becoming more widely accepted, many still follow the older step-up treatment modality. Siegel and colleagues strove to understand medication practices in a large US claims database study (28,119 patients with UC and 16,260 patients with CD) that examined patients from 2008 to 2016. Strikingly, in this study, less than 1% of patients with UC and less than 5% of patients with CD were treated first-line with biologics; instead, UC patients were most commonly started on 5-aminosalicylic acid monotherapy (61% of the patients), and patients with CD were started on corticosteroid monotherapy (42%).[10] One cause of this slow shift to adopting early effective therapy strategies is that "step-up" therapy has been extensively used by insurance companies to deny provider-selected therapies. A 2016 survey by the Crohn's and Colitis Foundation found that 40% of patients were forced by their insurance company to follow step therapy against their provider's advice.[11]

Benefits of Early Effective Therapy in Crohn's Disease

Analyses of clinical trial data have reported superior clinical outcomes in patients with CD with shorter disease duration. A post-hoc analysis of the PRECiSE 2 study of certolizumab-pegol in moderate-to-severe CD showed that those with treatment within a year of diagnosis had a 90% response rate compared to a 57% response rate in those diagnosed 5 years or more prior to therapy.[12] A similar post-hoc analysis of the CHARM trial, which was the trial of adalimumab (ADA) for maintenance therapy for adult, moderate-to-severe CD, showed numerically improved remission rates in patients with disease duration less than 2 years (43%) compared to two longer duration cohorts (2–5 years: 30%; >5 years: 28%).[13] A post-hoc analysis of CALM, a trial examining anti-TNF escalation in the setting of tight disease monitoring, studied long-term outcomes in the patients who were diagnosed early (n = 122, 50% of CALM; median 0.2 years from diagnosis); they found that, when deep remission is achieved in these early patients, they had an 81% decrease in adverse outcomes to 3 years.[14] Beyond anti-TNF, a retrospective review of the VICTORY consortium showed that patients with CD with disease duration of 2 years or less had improved response to vedolizumab therapy.[15] Similarly, LOVE-CD, which examined response to vedolizumab in early (<2 years from diagnosis) and late CD (>2 years from diagnosis), showed that endoscopic remission (SES-CD = 0: Early: 45%, Late: 15%, P = .0001) and combined steroid-free clinical remission and endoscopic remission (CDAI<150 + SES-CD ≤3: Early: 47%, Late: 16%, P = .0001) were both significantly better in the early cohort treated with vedolizumab.[16]

The benefits of early therapy have also been examined in prospective randomized controlled trials (RCT). One such trial randomized patients newly-diagnosed with CD to either early initiation of combination therapy with infliximab and thiopurine to initiation of thiopurine alone. Early infliximab therapy led to nearly two-thirds (62%) achieving clinical remission at 1 year compared to less than half (42%) on thiopurine alone.[17] This was further examined in the Randomized Evaluation of an Algorithm for Crohn's Treatment (REACT-1) cluster RCT (n = 1982) which looked not at initiation after diagnosis but an accelerated version of step-up therapy.[18] Serious complication and need for hospital admission or surgery were reduced in those who were using the accelerated model.[18]

There is also pediatric specific data that supports improvements in outcomes for early therapy with a biologic. Within RISK, a large (n = 1813) inception cohort of pediatric patients with CD, early treatment with anti-TNF was superior to early treatment with an immunomodulator in achieving remission at 1 year (85.3% vs 60.3%; Relative Risk: 1.41 [95% CI: 1.14–1.75]; P = .0017). Linear growth was also noted to be improved only in the early anti-TNFα group.[19] This was shown again in a small study (n = 31) from South Korea where relapse rates were improved in those who received infliximab just after diagnosis compared to those who started infliximab after failing conventional therapy with azathioprine and mesalamine (21% improvement in infliximab at diagnosis group in relapse-free rates at 3 years, P = .0094). Multivariable analysis from this small study revealed that the duration from the initial diagnosis to infliximab infusion was the only factor associated with relapse-free remission at 3 years (Hazard Ratio (HR): 1.077 [95% CI: 1.025–1.131]).[20] The data had been retrospective in nature, but a recently-published, multicenter, randomized trial from three European countries (the Netherlands, Finland, and Croatia) that enrolled 100 pediatric patients with CD showed again that first-line infliximab led to improvements in short-term endoscopic remission at 10 weeks (59% vs 17%, P = .001), long-term remission without escalation at 52 weeks (41% vs 15%; P = .004), and growth (Median change in SD score: +0.09 vs −0.13, P = .020), lending even more compelling support for the use of early effective therapy with biologics in pediatric patients with IBD.[21]

Benefits of Early Effective Therapy in Ulcerative Colitis

Within UC, the data does not compellingly support early effective therapy. In a cohort of 213 patients with UC treated with anti-TNF, Murthy and colleagues showed that longer disease duration was associated with higher 1-year steroid free remission (adjusted odds ratio (OR) = 2.1 [95% CI: 1.2–3.5] per 10-year increase in disease duration, P = .061) and a lower risk of colectomy (adjusted HR = 0.49 [95% CI: 0.28–0.85] per 10-year increase, P = .0048).[22] Mandel and colleagues similarly did not reveal a benefit of early anti-TNF exposure (within 3 years from diagnosis) in a cohort of 42 patients with UC.[23] Cases of acute severe UC, characterized by the onset of rapid and severe disease, carry a high risk of colectomy and may complicate these analyses.[24]

For therapies other than anti-TNF, the retrospective review of the VICTORY consortium did not show improvement in response to vedolizumab in patients with UC with shorter disease durations.[15] This was confirmed in the LOVE-UC Study, which looked at response to vedolizumab in early (<4 years disease duration) versus late (>4 years disease duration) UC, where they showed no difference in remission rates at week 26 between these two groups (Early: 49%; Late: 43%).[25]

Pediatric data is nearly non-existent on this topic. There is one study of 121 children with UC that compared outcomes in children who were started on azathioprine early (within 6 months of diagnosis) versus late (between 6–24 months after diagnosis). They did not find any differences in rates of surgery, hospitalization, treatment escalation, disease extension, or episodes of acute severe colitis between these two groups.[26] Thus, the available literature is retrospective, primarily adult, but it does consistently support that, in UC, there is no clear benefit for early therapy. There is an active European prospective trial (SPRINT, EudraCT number: 2020–003420–16) aiming to more cleanly examine the benefits of early therapy in adult UC, but pediatric trials remain much-needed.

Debating the Definition of Early

It should also be noted that there remains disagreement about the definition of early IBD. Two years from diagnosis has been suggested by some experts,[27] but this is very different from other diseases, like rheumatoid arthritis (RA), where much shorter intervals are described (eg, 3 months in RA).[28] The long delays in diagnosis in IBD further affect this definition as 2 years after diagnosis may translate to 5 years after occult disease onset.[29,30]

THE RIGHT PATIENT: PROGNOSTICATION

To pair the right therapy with the right patient right away, defining the prognosis of the patient is critical. In current clinical practice, prognosis is most commonly determined by combining clinical factors with traditional laboratory markers. At times, some may incorporate serologic responses to enteric pathogens and auto-antigens. There is also a burgeoning body of research looking to expand these prognostic markers.[31]

Clinical Factors

Within pediatrics, all patients are inherently diagnosed in a pediatric age range, and it has commonly been noted in both UC and CD that a younger age of diagnosis is associated with increased risk of relapses and recurrences.[32–35] Beyond age of diagnosis and the paired characteristic of disease duration, disease location or extent have also been tied to worsened outcomes. Perianal, ileocolonic, and upper tract disease phenotypes are associated with a more severe disease course in CD,[34–36] and, in UC, extensive colitis carries a higher colectomy risk.[37] Progressive disease, either with complication in CD[38–40] or extension in UC,[33,41] has also been shown to predict negative outcomes.

Worse prognosis is also tied to extraintestinal manifestations (EIM) and/or concomitant immune-mediated inflammatory diseases (IMIDs). EIM are thought to represent a sizable systemic inflammatory burden, and it is not surprising that they correlate with a worsened disease course.[42] A systematic review of 93 studies identified that patients with IBD and another IMID carried a higher risk for extensive colitis/pancolitis and IBD-related surgeries (Extensive/pancolitis: risk ratio [RR] 1.38; 95% CI 1.25, 1.52; $P < .01$, $I^2 = 86\%$; IBD-related surgeries: RR 1.17; 95% CI 1.01,1.36; $P = .03$; $I^2 = 85\%$).[43] Another study similarly found on multivariate analysis that patients diagnosed with an IMID prior to the onset of IBD carried an increased surgical risk (OR 3.71; 95% CI 2.1–6.56), leading them to conclude a pre-existing IMID was a poor prognostic factor in patients with IBD.[44]

Clinically-Available Proteomics

Two classic markers in IBD are C-reactive protein (CRP) and fecal calprotectin (FC), and, while they are primarily markers of disease activity, they have been tied to disease prognosis. Elevations in CRP have been tied to an increased need for surgery in both CD and UC,[45] and this can be true even in the face of clinical remission in CD.[46] However, there are issues with sensitivity and specificity for intestinal inflammation with CRP, and FC improves upon this.[47] In fact, serial measurements of FC have been shown to predict disease progression/relapse.[48–50] Both serologic responses to enteric pathogens and autoantigens, like anti-*Saccharomyces cerevisiae* antibody (ASCA), antibody to flagellin (CBir1), granulocyte-macrophage colony-stimulating factor (GMCSF), and perinuclear antineutrophil antibody (pANCA), have been implicated in prediction of IBD. In a large prospective study of pediatric patients with CD, being positive for a greater number of antimicrobial antigens was associated with a faster progression to complicated disease.[7] A number of studies have found that high expression of GMCSF autoantibodies is associated with complicated CD.[51–53] Intriguingly, these antibodies have also been shown to rise prior to disease inception in pre-diagnosis serum from military servicemen in PREDICTS (PRoteomic Evaluation and Discovery in an IBD Cohort of Tri-service Subjects).[54]

Predictive Biomarkers on the Horizon

There are numerous predictive markers on the horizon running the 'omic gamut.[31] RISK and PROTECT, pediatric inception cohorts of CD and UC respectively, have both identified transcriptomic signatures associated with prognosis. RISK found an extracellular matrix tissue transcriptomic signature present at diagnosis that could predict stricturing within 3 years of follow-up; they also combined this signature with other clinical and serologic markers to make a comprehensive risk model that still requires validation.[7] RISK has validated another transcriptomic module, which was derived from cells from the lamina propria, associated with failure to achieve durable remission.[55] The PROTECT cohort identified two predictive gene signatures – one for severity and another for therapeutic response; these signatures implicated lymphocyte activation, cytokine signaling, and mitochondrial dysfunction in UC, and they also warrant validation.[56] There is currently only one validated prognostic blood test; this is a CD8+ T cell gene expression profiling panel that places patients with IBD into low- and high-risk groups[57]; notably, steroid use can impact the results, which may affect its clinical utility.[58]

Regarding genomics, one large genome wide association study identified four loci linked to prognosis (*FOXO3*, *XACT*, a region near *IGFBP1*, and large parts of the MHC) that were *distinct* from susceptibility loci, indicating a role for different risk variants in prognosis than in diagnosis.[59] Polygenic risk scores and polymorphisms of nucleotide-binding oligomerization domain 2 (*NOD2*) have also been examined in prognosis, but, in pediatrics, within the RISK cohort, neither a PRS nor NOD2 were associated with stricturing or fistulizing behavior in CD.[7] Techniques to optimize genome-wide polygenic risk scores do continue to improve as more sophisticated techniques are incorporated, and they warrant further study.[60] Also in a more nascent phase, microbiome, metabolomic, and glycomic signatures are all still being developed in numerous studies to inform prognosis in IBD.[61–65] Network-based methods can also bridge the gap between all these multi'omic data, allowing for the integration of gene regulatory networks, protein-protein interactions, and microbiome-metabolomic networks[66–68]; creation of these networks could aid identification of a patient's personalized disease subtype and the ideal therapy or therapies for that subtype.

THE RIGHT DRUG: SEQUENCING & OTHER DRIVERS OF THERAPEUTIC CHOICE
The First-Line Therapy

Unfortunately, making a data-driven decision about first-line therapy has been historically difficult due to a dearth of head-to-head comparative trials. This has been recognized, and head-to-head comparisons are becoming more common. The first such ground-breaking trial, VARSITY, was published in 2019, and it compared patients with UC (n = 769) treated with either vedolizumab or adalimumab; 1-year outcomes were significantly improved in those treated with vedolizumab (clinical remission: VDZ 39%, ADA 23%, P = .006; endoscopic improvement: VDZ 40%, ADA 28%, P < .001).[69] Last year brought SEAVUE, the next such head-to-head comparison of ustekinumab and adalimumab in patients with CD (n = 386), and it showed no significant differences between the two therapies (P = .47); yet, there was a trend to improved endoscopic response in those on ustekinumab.[70] Another set of trials were also recently presented comparing etrolizumab to infliximab[71] and adalimumab[72] without significant differences between the therapeis. Finally, guselkumab, an IL-23 blocker, was recently compared to ustekinumab, an IL-12/23 blocker, to assess the differential effect using slightly more targeted blockade and, while it did not reveal significant differences, this could be due to an issue of power.[73]

Does the Order Matter?

As these new therapies have entered the IBD armamentarium, there is increased urgency to understand the impact of the sequence of therapies to better understand how to position them. Response to first-line therapy still remains relatively low; in one large study, approximately one-third of patients remained on the first-line biologic during the follow-up period while the other two-thirds changed to another therapy.[74] Most of the data on newer therapies examines their effect in the setting of failure, both primary and secondary, to anti-TNF therapies. As such, it has been observed that second-line and beyond therapies commonly have a decrease in efficacy/effectiveness,[75,76] underlining the importance of the choice of the first-line therapy.

Regarding the choice of the second-line and beyond therapies, there are several studies examining vedolizumab and ustekinumab after inadequate or loss of response to anti-TNF. Two of these studies supported superiority of ustekinumab over vedolizumab when used after anti-TNF.[77,78] Interestingly, another study reported no significant difference between the two medications when used *third-line* after anti-TNF and then either vedolizumab or ustekinumab.[79] Interestingly, there is some developing data from anti-IL23 medications, like risankizumab, mirikizumab, and guselkumab, that they do not have diminished effectiveness in those failing prior biologics lending support to the concept of improved effectiveness of this pathway post failure of another biologic.[80–82] It has been shown that anti-TNF non-responders had upregulation of IL23p19, IL23 R, and IL17 A, hinting at a biological explanation for these observations.[83]

Furthermore, Kugathasan and colleagues found significantly higher levels of IL12p40 and IL12 Rβ2 messenger RNA and INF-γ production by T cells in children with early compared with late CD. This had led to speculation that IL-12 may be an important pathway in early disease as well as anti-TNF refractory disease, and therapies targeting this pathway should be moved earlier in treatment algorithms.[84]

There is also mounting evidence that JAK inhibitors may maintain effectiveness after biologic failure with both tofacitinib and upadacitinib demonstrating significant effectiveness even in patients with history of inadequate or loss of response to prior biologic therapies.[85,86] This may in part be the result of overcoming issues of clearance since small molecule therapies are not cleared in the same way as biologic therapies; however, their success is certainly more complex than just through enhancement of clearance, since another group of small molecules, selective sphingosine 1-phosphate receptor modulators, do not fare as well in patients with multiple biologic failures.[87]

Finally, it has been proposed that rational early use of combinations of therapies may be a route to enhance response and remission rates by targeting complementary biological pathways. The Study of Biologic and Immunomodulator Naive Patients in Crohn's Disease (SONIC) famously described the superiority of the combination of thiopurine and anti-TNF, and this led to its commonplace use.[88] When it was elucidated that the benefit came from decreasing immunogenicity and enhancing bioavailability,[89] this combination has fallen out of favor, particularly in pediatrics, as optimized monotherapy allows avoidance of the adverse effects of thiopurine.[90] There is some observational data on the use of other types of combinations in both adults[91] and pediatrics,[92] but more data needs to be generated on the efficacy and safety of this approach. One such randomized controlled trial, the VEGA trial (n = 214), compared the combination use of golimumab and guselkumab to their individual use as monotherapy for moderate-to-severe UC. Endoscopic improvement was more likely in those on combination compared with either monotherapy (golimumab: P = .003; guselkumab: P = .016), and adverse events were not higher with combination.[93,94] Another study, EXPLORER, examined the combination of vedolizumab, adalimumab, and methotrexate in bio-naïve patients with CD at high risk for complications; at 26 weeks, 35% were in endoscopic remission, 55% were in clinical remission, and 11% had serious adverse events, which supports the safety of this combination but did not lead to the desired large delta in outcomes.[93]

Beyond medical therapies, there are certain clinical scenarios in CD where surgery may be the appropriate initial choice of treatment. The LIR!C trial, a randomized trial of adult patients with CD, showed no difference in clinical outcomes, both remission and quality-of-life, between anti-TNF biologic medication and ileocecal resection,[95] even in longer-term follow-up for over 5 years.[96] Pediatric data is limited in this area, and it warrants further investigation. It should be noted that high-volume centers lead to fewer complications for both adult and pediatric patients with IBD, making the availability of skilled surgeons an important factor to consider when positioning surgery.[97,98]

Two Immune-Mediated Inflammatory Diseases, One Treatment

In addition to impacting prognosis, EIMs and concomitant IMIDs can also inform treatment choices.

Various types of articular issues affect patients with IBD.[99] When a patient has significant joint involvement, anti-TNF is often considered the therapy of choice, supported by clinical trial data.[100,101] Conversely, patients treated with vedolizumab have been shown to have an increased incidence of joint extraintestinal manifestation compared to patients treated with anti-TNF[102]; however, there is still some potential to improve peripheral arthritis in vedolizumab by reducing overall disease activity.[103]

Dermatologic manifestations are also common in IBD.[99] Patients with pre-existing atopic dermatitis may experience a worsening on anti-TNF therapies,[104] and newer therapies like upadacitinib carry dual approvals for UC and atopic dermatitis.[105] Similarly, psoriasis or a psoriasiform dermatitis in patients with IBD may benefit from a change to a medication that blocks IL12 and/or IL23.[104]

There are some limitations in data on the choice of therapy to best manage perianal fistula. Infliximab is the current therapy of choice as it is the only medication supported by an RCT (n = 366) to improve fistula closure (36% vs 19% with placebo).[106] There are, however, some promising post-hoc sub-group analyses and retrospective studies of adalimumab,[107] ustekinumab,[108] and vedolizumab.[109] Additionally, the choice of drug may not be the only important choice for perianal fistulae since the dose is also very important; studies have shown that achieving high drug concentrations leads to improved fistula closure.[110]

Predicting Safety: Pharmacogenomics & Family History

Choosing therapy consists not only of predicting efficacy but also reducing adverse events. Pharmacogenomics has a role in predicting safety of thiopurine and anti-TNF therapies. For thiopurines, in the 1980s, variants of the thiopurine methyltransferase (TPMT) gene were found to be associated with decreased enzymatic activity that could result in severe leukopenia. More recently, mutations in Nudix hydrolase (NUDT15) were also identified as impacting leukopenia risk.[111,112] Patients with a combination of TPMT and NUDT15 risk variants represented ~50% of those suffering severe thiopurine-induced leukopenia in one study,[112] and, as such, it is recommended to check for these variants prior to initiating thiopurine therapy.[113]

Risk variants impacting biologic therapies are less common, and there is only one used currently in clinical practice. This variant, HLA-DQA1*05, was identified by the Personalizing Anti-TNF Therapy in CD (PANTS) consortium (n = 1240), and they presented that it significantly increased the risk of developing anti-drug antibodies to anti-TNF therapies (HR 1.90, 95% CI: 1.60–2.25).[114] This finding has been replicated in several other cohorts, with the risk variant present in an average of 43% of patients with IBD across 14 studies and a meta-analysis of this data confirming the increase risk of immunogenicity (OR 1.63, 95% CI: 1.35–1.98).[115] However, the clinical utility of this variant appears to depend on the strategy of therapeutic drug monitoring, with variant carriers in two primarily pediatric cohorts using proactive monitoring *not* at increased risk for anti-drug antibodies.[116,117] Discovery should continue to identify potential risk variants for newer therapies to better develop a broad pharmacogenomic assessment that may guide treatment selection, like that which exists for psychiatric medications.[118]

Cost: a Primary Driver of Treatment Selection

Given the high cost of the specialty medications used in IBD, there is a tension between the cost of therapy and the benefit to the patient. The COIN study in the Netherlands reported in 2014 that biologics accounted for 64% and 31% of the total cost for CD and UC respectively.[119] Pillai and colleagues investigated the effectiveness of early biologic use and found, when using the cost of originator infliximab, it was not cost effective. However, a reduction in cost of therapy by 30% led to improvements in cost-effectiveness for early therapy.[120] Biosimilars have been shown to reduce costs by 15% to 35%, which may tilt the scales in favor of early therapy.[121] Early surgery in a randomized trial of adult patients with CD has also been shown to be a cost-effective option, but, again, pediatric data is limited.[122]

In an intriguing analysis within UC, Bloudek and colleagues modeled 21 sequences of therapies. They found the sequence that optimized net health benefits and minimized costs started with infliximab or biosimilars as the first-line treatment and then moved to tofacitinib, adalimumab, or vedolizumab as next line. Interestingly, when quality-adjusted life-years (QALY) were maximized, removing the emphasis on minimization of costs, ustekinumab followed by vedolizumab was the top-ranked sequence.[123]

Patient Preference & Shared Decision Making

Finally, as more therapies are available, patients have more ability to weigh in on their therapeutic choice if they desire.[124] In a large telephone survey, patients with both UC and CD rated effectiveness as the most important factor they weighed, but frequency of serious adverse events and mode of administration also were highly relevant.[125] Patients tend to be more likely to choose SC administration over IV infusion, but individual preferences vary.[126,127] Shared decision making with patients is, thus, becoming even more vital. Providers need to identify how much input the patient wants to provide and then arm the patient with enough education to weigh their options. When a patient can collaborate in their plan of care, they are more confident in their choice and more adherent to therapy, which can lead to improved outcomes.[124]

SUMMARY

Choosing the right therapy in IBD requires weighing factors as heterogenous as the disease itself. The best drug should be one matched to the patient's key inflammatory pathway(s) to achieve the highest possible efficacy; it should also maximize safety, given the need for long-term use particularly in pediatrics. Ideally, it should also be identified upfront to minimize the accrual of bowel wall damage and any impact on efficacy of prior inefficacious therapies. On top of all this, the decision must take into account factors as varied as concomitant immune-mediated inflammatory diseases, patient preferences, and costs. While it remains a delicate balancing act to identify these "rights," this review has presented how they can be practically carried out in the clinic right now.

CLINICS CARE POINTS

- Precision Medicine can be currently accomplished in the clinic through targeted treatment choice using clinical characteristics (e.g. severe phenotype, EIM, concomitant IMID) and pharmacogenomics.

- Patients should be involved in the treatment decision through the consideration of patient preferences in addition to clinical factors.

- Early effective therapy is beneficial in CD, and, in IBD broadly, first therapies are often markedly superior to subsequent therapies; thus, maximizing the potential effectiveness of the first therapy is vital for all patients with IBD.

DISCLOSURES

E.A. Spencer is supported by a grant from the NIH, United States (K23DK125760-01). E.A. Spencer has served on an advisory board for Prometheus Laboratories, Inc.

REFERENCES

1. Alsoud D, Verstockt B, Fiocchi C, et al. Breaking the therapeutic ceiling in drug development in ulcerative colitis. The lancet Gastroenterology & hepatology 2021;6(7):589–95.

2. Spencer EA, Dubinsky MC. Precision Medicine in Pediatric Inflammatory Bowel Disease. Pediatric Clinics 2021;68(6):1171–90.

3. Torres J, Mehandru S, Colombel JF, et al. Crohn's disease. Lancet 2017; 389(10080):1741–55.

4. Ungaro R, Mehandru S, Allen PB, et al. Ulcerative colitis. Lancet 2017; 389(10080):1756–70.

5. Agrawal M, Spencer EA, Colombel J-F, et al. Approach to the Management of Recently Diagnosed Inflammatory Bowel Disease Patients: A User's Guide for Adult and Pediatric Gastroenterologists. Gastroenterology 2021;161(1):47–65.

6. Pigneur B, Seksik P, Viola S, et al. Natural history of Crohn's disease: Comparison between childhood- and adult-onset disease. Inflamm Bowel Dis 2010; 16(6):953–61.

7. Kugathasan S, Denson LA, Walters TD, et al. Prediction of complicated disease course for children newly diagnosed with Crohn's disease: a multicentre inception cohort study. Lancet 2017;389(10080):1710–8.

8. Torres J, Billioud V, Sachar DB, et al. Ulcerative colitis as a progressive disease: the forgotten evidence. Inflamm Bowel Dis 2012;18(7):1356–63.

9. Danese S, Fiorino G, Fernandes C, et al. Catching the therapeutic window of opportunity in early Crohn's disease. Curr Drug Targets 2014;15(11):1056–63.

10. Siegel CA, Yang F, Eslava S, et al. Treatment Pathways Leading to Biologic Therapies for Ulcerative Colitis and Crohn's Disease in the United States. Clin Transl Gastroenterol 2020;11(2).

11. Rubin DT, Feld LD, Goeppinger SR, et al. The Crohn's and Colitis Foundation of America Survey of Inflammatory Bowel Disease Patient Health Care Access. Inflamm Bowel Dis 2017;23(2):224–32.

12. Schreiber S, Colombel JF, Bloomfield R, et al. Increased response and remission rates in short-duration Crohn's disease with subcutaneous certolizumab pegol: an analysis of PRECiSE 2 randomized maintenance trial data. Am J Gastroenterol 2010;105(7):1574–82.

13. Schreiber S, Reinisch W, Colombel JF, et al. Subgroup analysis of the placebo-controlled CHARM trial: increased remission rates through 3 years for adalimumab-treated patients with early Crohn's disease. J Crohns Colitis 2013;7(3):213–21.

14. Ungaro RC, Yzet C, Bossuyt P, et al. Deep Remission at 1 Year Prevents Progression of Early Crohn's Disease. Gastroenterology 2020. https://doi.org/10. 1053/j.gastro.2020.03.039.

15. Faleck DM, Winters A, Chablaney S, et al. Shorter Disease Duration Is Associated With Higher Rates of Response to Vedolizumab in Patients With Crohn's Disease But Not Ulcerative Colitis. Clin Gastroenterol Hepatol 2019;17(12): 2497–505.e1. https://doi.org/10.1016/j.cgh.2018.12.040.

16. D'Haens GR, Bossuyt P, Baert F, et al. Higher endoscopic AND clinical remission rates with vedolizumab in early than in late crohn's disease: results from the Love-Cd study (low countries vedolizumab in Cd study). presented at. Vienna: UEGW; 2022. Session OP130.

17. D'Haens G, Baert F, van Assche G, et al. Early combined immunosuppression or conventional management in patients with newly diagnosed Crohn's disease: an open randomised trial. Lancet 2008;371(9613):660–7.

18. Khanna R, Bressler B, Levesque BG, et al. Early combined immunosuppression for the management of Crohn's disease (REACT): a cluster randomised controlled trial. Lancet 2015;386(10006):1825–34.

19. Walters TD, Kim M-O, Denson LA, et al. Increased Effectiveness of Early Therapy With Anti-Tumor Necrosis Factor-α vs an Immunomodulator in Children With Crohn's Disease. *Gastroenterology.* 2014;146(2):383-391. doi:10.1053/j.gastro.2013.10.027.

20. Lee YM, Kang B, Lee Y, et al. Infliximab "Top-Down" Strategy is Superior to "Step-Up" in Maintaining Long-Term Remission in the Treatment of Pediatric Crohn Disease. J Pediatr Gastroenterol Nutr 2015;60(6).

21. Jongsma MME, Aardoom MA, Cozijnsen MA, et al. First-line treatment with infliximab versus conventional treatment in children with newly diagnosed moderate-to-severe Crohn's disease: an open-label multicentre randomised controlled trial. Gut 2022;71(1):34–42.

22. Murthy SK, Greenberg GR, Croitoru K, et al. Extent of Early Clinical Response to Infliximab Predicts Long-term Treatment Success in Active Ulcerative Colitis. Inflamm Bowel Dis 2015;21(9):2090–6.

23. Mandel MD, Balint A, Golovics PA, et al. Decreasing trends in hospitalizations during anti-TNF therapy are associated with time to anti-TNF therapy: Results from two referral centres. Dig Liver Dis 2014;46(11):985–90.

24. Dulai PS, Jairath V. Acute severe ulcerative colitis: latest evidence and therapeutic implications. Ther Adv Chronic Dis 2018;9(2):65–72.

25. Vermeire S, Löwenberg M, Ferrante M, et al. 456 Efficacy, safety and mucosal healing of early versus late use of vedolizumab in ulcerative colitis: results from the love-uc study. Gastroenterology 2021;160(6). S-91-S-92.

26. Aloi M, D'Arcangelo G, Bramuzzo M, et al. Effect of Early Versus Late Azathioprine Therapy in Pediatric Ulcerative Colitis. Inflamm Bowel Dis 2016;22(7):1647–54.

27. Peyrin-Biroulet L, Loftus EV Jr, Colombel JF, et al. Early Crohn disease: a proposed definition for use in disease-modification trials. Gut 2010;59(2):141–7.

28. Nell VP, Machold KP, Eberl G, et al. Benefit of very early referral and very early therapy with disease-modifying anti-rheumatic drugs in patients with early rheumatoid arthritis. Rheumatology 2004;43(7):906–14.

29. Sulkanen E, Repo M, Huhtala H, et al. Impact of diagnostic delay to the clinical presentation and associated factors in pediatric inflammatory bowel disease: a retrospective study. BMC Gastroenterol 2021;21(1):364.

30. Gallinger Z, Ungaro R, Colombel J-F, Sandler RS, Chen W. P030 Delayed diagnosis of crohn's disease is common and associated with an increased risk of disease complications. *Gastroenterology.* 2019;156(3):S21. doi:10.1053/j.gastro.2019.01.081.

31. Verstockt B, Noor NM, Marigorta UM, et al. Results of the Seventh Scientific Workshop of ECCO: Precision Medicine in IBD—Disease Outcome and Response to Therapy. Journal of Crohn's and Colitis 2021;15(9):1431–42.

32. Roth LS, Chande N, Ponich T, et al. Predictors of disease severity in ulcerative colitis patients from Southwestern Ontario. World J Gastroenterol 2010;16(2):232–6.

33. Etchevers MJ, Aceituno M, García-Bosch O, et al. Risk factors and characteristics of extent progression in ulcerative colitis. Inflamm Bowel Dis 2009;15(9):1320–5.

34. Solberg IC, Lygren I, Jahnsen J, et al. Clinical course during the first 10 years of ulcerative colitis: results from a population-based inception cohort (IBSEN Study). Scand J Gastroenterol 2009;44(4):431–40.

35. Beaugerie L, Seksik P, Nion-Larmurier I, et al. Predictors of Crohn's disease. Gastroenterology 2006;130(3):650–6.

36. Torres J, Caprioli F, Katsanos KH, et al. Predicting Outcomes to Optimize Disease Management in Inflammatory Bowel Diseases. Journal of Crohn's & colitis 2016;10(12):1385–94.
37. Ulcerative Colitis Clinical Care Pathway. https://s3.amazonaws.com/agaassets/pdf/guidelines/UlcerativeColitis/index.html.
38. Siegel CA, Whitman CB, Spiegel BMR, et al. Development of an index to define overall disease severity in IBD. Gut 2018;67(2):244–54.
39. AGA institute guidelines for the Identification, Assessment and Initial Medical Treatment in Crohn's Disease: Clinical Decision Support Tool. https://s3.amazonaws.com/agaassets/pdf/guidelines/IBDCarePathway.pdf.
40. Zhao M, Lo BZS, Vester-Andersen MK, et al. A 10-Year Follow-up Study of the Natural History of Perianal Crohn's Disease in a Danish Population-Based Inception Cohort. Inflamm Bowel Dis 2019;25(7):1227–36. https://doi.org/10.1093/ibd/izy374.
41. Qiu Y, Chen B, Li Y, et al. Risk factors and long-term outcome of disease extent progression in Asian patients with ulcerative colitis: a retrospective cohort study. BMC Gastroenterol 2019;19(1):7.
42. Veloso FT. Extraintestinal manifestations of inflammatory bowel disease: do they influence treatment and outcome? World J Gastroenterol 2011;17(22):2702–7.
43. Attauabi M, Zhao M, Bendtsen F, et al. Systematic Review with Meta-analysis: The Impact of Co-occurring Immune-mediated Inflammatory Diseases on the Disease Course of Inflammatory Bowel Diseases. Inflamm Bowel Dis 2020. https://doi.org/10.1093/ibd/izaa167.
44. García MJ, Pascual M, Del Pozo C, et al. Impact of immune-mediated diseases in inflammatory bowel disease and implications in therapeutic approach. Sci Rep 2020;10(1):10731.
45. Henriksen M, Jahnsen J, Lygren I, et al. C-reactive protein: a predictive factor and marker of inflammation in inflammatory bowel disease. Results from a prospective population-based study. Gut 2008;57(11):1518–23.
46. Oh K, Oh EH, Baek S, et al. Elevated C-reactive protein level during clinical remission can predict poor outcomes in patients with Crohn's disease. PLoS One 2017;12(6):e0179266.
47. Sands BE. Biomarkers of Inflammation in Inflammatory Bowel Disease. Gastroenterology 2015;149(5):1275–85.e2.
48. Park J, Yoon H, Shin CM, et al. Clinical factors to predict flare-up in patients with inflammatory bowel disease during international air travel: A prospective study. PLoS One 2022;17(1):e0262571.
49. De Vos M, Louis EJ, Jahnsen J, et al. Consecutive fecal calprotectin measurements to predict relapse in patients with ulcerative colitis receiving infliximab maintenance therapy. Inflamm Bowel Dis 2013;19(10):2111–7.
50. Kennedy NA, Jones G-R, Plevris N, et al. Association Between Level of Fecal Calprotectin and Progression of Crohn's Disease. Clin Gastroenterol Hepatol 2019;17(11):2269–76.e4. https://doi.org/10.1016/j.cgh.2019.02.017.
51. Gathungu G, Kim MO, Ferguson JP, et al. Granulocyte-macrophage colony-stimulating factor autoantibodies: a marker of aggressive Crohn's disease. Inflamm Bowel Dis 2013;19(8):1671–80.
52. Han X, Uchida K, Jurickova I, et al. Granulocyte-macrophage colony-stimulating factor autoantibodies in murine ileitis and progressive ileal Crohn's disease. Gastroenterology 2009;136(4):1261–71, e1-e3.
53. Mortha A, Remark R, Del Valle DM, et al. Neutralizing Anti-Granulocyte Macrophage-Colony Stimulating Factor Autoantibodies Recognize Post-Translational

Glycosylations on Granulocyte Macrophage-Colony Stimulating Factor Years Before Diagnosis and Predict Complicated Crohn's Disease. Gastroenterology 2022;163(3):659–70.

54. Choung RS, Princen F, Stockfisch TP, et al. Serologic microbial associated markers can predict Crohn's disease behaviour years before disease diagnosis. Aliment Pharmacol Ther 2016;43(12):1300–10.

55. Martin JC, Chang C, Boschetti G, et al. Single-Cell Analysis of Crohn's Disease Lesions Identifies a Pathogenic Cellular Module Associated with Resistance to Anti-TNF Therapy. Cell 2019;178(6):1493–508.e20.

56. Haberman Y, Karns R, Dexheimer PJ, et al. Ulcerative colitis mucosal transcriptomes reveal mitochondriopathy and personalized mechanisms underlying disease severity and treatment response. Nat Commun 2019;10(1):38.

57. Biasci D, Lee JC, Noor NM, et al. A blood-based prognostic biomarker in IBD. Gut 2019;68(8):1386–95.

58. Alsoud D, Verstockt S, Sabino J, et al. P062 Effects of exposure to steroids on the PredictSURE whole blood prognostic assay in Inflammatory Bowel Disease. Journal of Crohn's and Colitis 2021;15(Supplement_1):S168.

59. Lee JC, Biasci D, Roberts R, et al. Genome-wide association study identifies distinct genetic contributions to prognosis and susceptibility in Crohn's disease. Nat Genet 2017;49(2):262–8.

60. Khera AV, Chaffin M, Aragam KG, et al. Genome-wide polygenic scores for common diseases identify individuals with risk equivalent to monogenic mutations. Nat Genet 2018;50(9):1219–24.

61. Keshteli AH, van den Brand FF, Madsen KL, et al. Dietary and metabolomic determinants of relapse in ulcerative colitis patients: A pilot prospective cohort study. World J Gastroenterol 2017;23(21):3890–9.

62. Hisamatsu T, Ono N, Imaizumi A, et al. Decreased Plasma Histidine Level Predicts Risk of Relapse in Patients with Ulcerative Colitis in Remission. PLoS One 2015;10(10):e0140716.

63. Britton GJ, Contijoch EJ, Mogno I, et al. Microbiotas from Humans with Inflammatory Bowel Disease Alter the Balance of Gut Th17 and RORγt(+) Regulatory T Cells and Exacerbate Colitis in Mice. Immunity 2019;50(1):212–24.e4.

64. Connelly MA, Otvos JD, Shalaurova I, et al. GlycA, a novel biomarker of systemic inflammation and cardiovascular disease risk. J Transl Med 2017;15(1):219.

65. Dierckx T, Verstockt B, Vermeire S, et al. GlycA, a Nuclear Magnetic Resonance Spectroscopy Measure for Protein Glycosylation, is a Viable Biomarker for Disease Activity in IBD. Journal of Crohn's and Colitis 2018;13(3):389–94.

66. Peters LA, Perrigoue J, Mortha A, et al. A functional genomics predictive network model identifies regulators of inflammatory bowel disease. Nat Genet 2017;49(10):1437–49.

67. Argmann C, Tokuyama M, Ungaro RC, et al. Molecular Characterization of Limited Ulcerative Colitis Reveals Novel Biology and Predictors of Disease Extension. Gastroenterology 2021;161(6):1953–68.e15.

68. Reiman D, Layden BT, Dai Y. MiMeNet: Exploring microbiome-metabolome relationships using neural networks. PLoS Comput Biol 2021;17(5):e1009021.

69. Sands BE, Peyrin-Biroulet L, Loftus EV Jr, et al. Vedolizumab versus Adalimumab for Moderate-to-Severe Ulcerative Colitis. N Engl J Med 2019;381(13):1215–26.

70. Sands BE, Irving PM, Hoops T, et al. Ustekinumab versus adalimumab for induction and maintenance therapy in biologic-naive patients with moderately to

severely active Crohn's disease: a multicentre, randomised, double-blind, parallel-group, phase 3b trial. Lancet 2022;399(10342):2200–11.

71. Danese S, Colombel J-F, Lukas M, et al. Etrolizumab versus infliximab for the treatment of moderately to severely active ulcerative colitis (GARDENIA): a randomised, double-blind, double-dummy, phase 3 study. The Lancet Gastroenterology & Hepatology 2022;7(2):118–27.

72. Rubin DT, Dotan I, DuVall A, et al. Etrolizumab versus adalimumab or placebo as induction therapy for moderately to severely active ulcerative colitis (HIBISCUS): two phase 3 randomised, controlled trials. The Lancet Gastroenterology & Hepatology 2022;7(1):17–27.

73. Sandborn WJ, D'Haens GR, Reinisch W, et al. Guselkumab for the Treatment of Crohn's Disease: Induction Results From the Phase 2 GALAXI-1 Study. *Gastroenterology*. 2022;162(6):1650-1664.e8. doi:10.1053/j.gastro.2022.01.047.

74. Brady JE, Stott-Miller M, Mu G, et al. Treatment Patterns and Sequencing in Patients With Inflammatory Bowel Disease. Clin Ther 2018;40(9):1509–21.e5.

75. Bressler B, Yarur A, Silverberg MS, et al. Vedolizumab and Anti-Tumour Necrosis Factor α Real-World Outcomes in Biologic-Naïve Inflammatory Bowel Disease Patients: Results from the EVOLVE Study. J Crohns Colitis 2021;15(10):1694–706.

76. Kassouri L, Amiot A, Kirchgesner J, et al. The outcome of Crohn's disease patients refractory to anti-TNF and either vedolizumab or ustekinumab. Dig Liver Dis 2020;52(10):1148–55.

77. Biemans VBC, van der Woude CJ, Dijkstra G, et al. Ustekinumab is associated with superior effectiveness outcomes compared to vedolizumab in Crohn's disease patients with prior failure to anti-TNF treatment. Aliment Pharmacol Ther 2020;52(1):123–34.

78. Alric H, Amiot A, Kirchgesner J, et al. The effectiveness of either ustekinumab or vedolizumab in 239 patients with Crohn's disease refractory to anti-tumour necrosis factor. Aliment Pharmacol Ther 2020;51(10):948–57.

79. Albshesh A, Taylor J, Savarino EV, et al. Effectiveness of Third-Class Biologic Treatment in Crohn's Disease: A Multi-Center Retrospective Cohort Study. J Clin Med 2021;10(13).

80. Ferrante M, Peyrin-Biroulet L, Dignass A, et al. Clinical and endoscopic improvements with risankizumab induction and maintenance dosing versus placebo are observed irrespective of number of prior failed biologics. Presented at: UEGW 2022; 2022; Vienna. Session S8. (Oral presentation at UEGW).

81. D'Haens GR, Kobayashi T, Morris N, Lissoos T, Hoover A, Sands B. Efficacy and safety of mirikizumab as induction therapy in patients with moderately to severely active ulcerative colitis: results from the phase 3 lucent-1 study. presented at: DDW 2022; 2022; San Diego Session S-214.

82. Panes J, Allegretti JR, Sands B, Huang KG, Kavalam M, Germinaro M. The effect of guselkumab induction therapy in patients with moderately to severely active ulcerative colitis: quasar phase 2b induction results at week 12 by prior inadequate response or intolerance to advanced therapy. presented at: UEGW; 2022; Vienna Session OP109.

83. Schmitt H, Billmeier U, Dieterich W, et al. Expansion of IL-23 receptor bearing TNFR2+ T cells is associated with molecular resistance to anti-TNF therapy in Crohn's disease. Gut 2019;68(5):814–28.

84. Kugathasan S, Saubermann LJ, Smith L, et al. Mucosal T-cell immunoregulation varies in early and late inflammatory bowel disease. Gut 2007;56(12):1696–705.

85. Loftus E Jr, Colombel JF, Lacerda AP, et al. Efficacy and safety of upadacitinib induction therapy in patients with moderately to severely active crohn's disease: results from a randomized phase 3 u-excel study. Vienna: UEGW; 2022. presented at.

86. Lee SD, Singla A, Harper J, et al. Tofacitinib Appears Well Tolerated and Effective for the Treatment of Patients with Refractory Crohn's Disease. Dig Dis Sci 2022;67(8):4043–8.

87. Feagan B, Peyrin-Biroulet L, Sandborn W, et al. Etrasimod 2mg once daily as treatment for biologic/janus kinase inhibitor-naïve and -experienced patients with moderately to severely active ulcerative colitis: subgroup analysis from the phase 3 elevate uc 52 and elevate uc 12 trials. Vienna: UEGW; 2022. presented at.

88. Colombel JF, Sandborn WJ, Reinisch W, et al. Infliximab, azathioprine, or combination therapy for Crohn's disease. N Engl J Med 2010;362(15):1383–95.

89. Mogensen DV, Brynskov J, Ainsworth MA, et al. A Role for Thiopurine Metabolites in the Synergism Between Thiopurines and Infliximab in Inflammatory Bowel Disease. Journal of Crohn's and Colitis 2017;12(3):298–305.

90. van Hoeve K, Vermeire S. Thiopurines in Pediatric Inflammatory Bowel Disease: Current and Future Place. Pediatr Drugs 2020;22(5):449–61.

91. Ahmed W, Galati J, Kumar A, et al. Dual Biologic or Small Molecule Therapy for Treatment of Inflammatory Bowel Disease: A Systematic Review and Meta-analysis. Clin Gastroenterol Hepatol 2022;20(3):e361–79.

92. Dolinger MT, Spencer EA, Lai J, et al. Dual Biologic and Small Molecule Therapy for the Treatment of Refractory Pediatric Inflammatory Bowel Disease. Inflamm Bowel Dis 2020. https://doi.org/10.1093/ibd/izaa277.

93. Colombel JF, Ungaro RC, Sands BE, et al. 885: Triple combination therapy with vedolizumab, adalimumab, and methotrexate in patients with high-risk crohn's disease: interim analysis from the open-label, phase 4 explorer trial. Gastroenterology 2022;162(7). S-215.

94. Panes J, Sands B, Sandborn WJ, et al. Induction combination therapy with guselkumab and golimumab followed by guselkumab monotherapy maintenance: results of the phase 2a, randomized, double-blind, proof-of-concept vega study. presented at. Vienna: UEGW; 2022. Session OP087.

95. Ponsioen CY, de Groof EJ, Eshuis EJ, et al. Laparoscopic ileocaecal resection versus infliximab for terminal ileitis in Crohn's disease: a randomised controlled, open-label, multicentre trial. The lancet Gastroenterology & hepatology 2017; 2(11):785–92.

96. Stevens TW, Haasnoot ML, D'Haens GR, et al. Laparoscopic ileocaecal resection versus infliximab for terminal ileitis in Crohn's disease: retrospective long-term follow-up of the LIR!C trial. The lancet Gastroenterology & hepatology 2020. https://doi.org/10.1016/S2468-1253(20)30117-5.

97. Egberg MD, Galanko JA, Kappelman MD. Patients Who Undergo Colectomy for Pediatric Ulcerative Colitis at Low-Volume Hospitals Have More Complications. Clin Gastroenterol Hepatol : the official clinical practice journal of the American Gastroenterological Association 2019;17(13):2713–21.e4.

98. Williams H, Alabbadi S, Egorova N, et al. Patients Undergoing Abdominal Operation for Crohn's Disease Have Lower Mortality and Readmission Rate at High-Volume Hospital Centers. J Am Coll Surg 2022;235(5).

99. Vavricka SR, Brun L, Ballabeni P, et al. Frequency and risk factors for extraintestinal manifestations in the Swiss inflammatory bowel disease cohort. Am J Gastroenterol 2011;106(1):110–9.

100. Herfarth H, Obermeier F, Andus T, et al. Improvement of arthritis and arthralgia after treatment with infliximab (Remicade) in a German prospective, open-label, multicenter trial in refractory Crohn's disease. Am J Gastroenterol 2002;97(10): 2688–90.

101. Louis EJ, Reinisch W, Schwartz DA, et al. Adalimumab Reduces Extraintestinal Manifestations in Patients with Crohn's Disease: A Pooled Analysis of 11 Clinical Studies. Adv Ther 2018;35(4):563–76.

102. Dubinsky MC, Cross RK, Sandborn WJ, et al. Extraintestinal Manifestations in Vedolizumab and Anti-TNF-Treated Patients With Inflammatory Bowel Disease. Inflamm Bowel Dis 2018;24(9):1876–82.

103. Kopylov U, Burisch J, Ben-Horin S, et al. P406 A retrospective analysis of the efficacy of vedolizumab on extra-intestinal manifestations in patients with inflammatory bowel disease across five European countries. Journal of Crohn's and Colitis 2021;15(Supplement_1):S412–4.

104. Dolinger MT, Rolfes P, Spencer E, et al. Outcomes of Children With Inflammatory Bowel Disease Who Develop Anti-Tumor Necrosis Factor Induced Skin Reactions. J Crohns Colitis 2022. https://doi.org/10.1093/ecco-jcc/jjac055.

105. Simpson EL, Papp KA, Blauvelt A, et al. Efficacy and Safety of Upadacitinib in Patients With Moderate to Severe Atopic Dermatitis: Analysis of Follow-up Data From the Measure Up 1 and Measure Up 2 Randomized Clinical Trials. JAMA Dermatology 2022;158(4):404–13.

106. Sands BE, Anderson FH, Bernstein CN, et al. Infliximab maintenance therapy for fistulizing Crohn's disease. N Engl J Med 2004;350(9):876–85.

107. Ruemmele FM, Rosh J, Faubion WA, et al. Efficacy of Adalimumab for Treatment of Perianal Fistula in Children with Moderately to Severely Active Crohn's Disease: Results from IMAgINE 1 and IMAgINE 2. J Crohns Colitis 2018;12(10): 1249–54.

108. Chapuis-Biron C, Kirchgesner J, Pariente B, et al. Ustekinumab for Perianal Crohn's Disease: The BioLAP Multicenter Study From the GETAID. Am J Gastroenterol 2020;115(11).

109. Tadbiri S, Grimaud JC, Peyrin-Biroulet L, et al. DOP025 Efficacy of vedolizumab on extraintestinal manifestation in patients with inflammatory bowel disease: a post-hoc analysis of the OBSERV-IBD cohort from the GETAID. J Crohn's Colitis 2017;11(suppl_1):S42.

110. Zulqarnain M, Deepak P, Yarur AJ. Therapeutic Drug Monitoring in Perianal Fistulizing Crohn's Disease. J Clin Med 2022;(7):11.

111. Moriyama T, Nishii R, Perez-Andreu V, et al. NUDT15 polymorphisms alter thiopurine metabolism and hematopoietic toxicity. Nat Genet 2016;48(4):367–73.

112. Schaeffeler E, Jaeger SU, Klumpp V, et al. Impact of NUDT15 genetics on severe thiopurine-related hematotoxicity in patients with European ancestry. Genet Med 2019;21(9):2145–50.

113. Feuerstein JD, Nguyen GC, Kupfer SS, et al. American Gastroenterological Association Institute Guideline on Therapeutic Drug Monitoring in Inflammatory Bowel Disease. Gastroenterology 2017;153(3):827–34.

114. Sazonovs A, Kennedy NA, Moutsianas L, et al. HLA-DQA1*05 Carriage Associated With Development of Anti-Drug Antibodies to Infliximab and Adalimumab in Patients With Crohn's Disease. Gastroenterology 2020;158(1):189–99.

115. Bergstein S, Spencer E. The association between the genetic variant HLA-DQA1*05 and the development of antibodies to anti-TNF therapy in the IBD population: a meta-analysis. 2022.

116. Spencer EA, Stachelski J, Dervieux T, et al. Failure to Achieve Target Drug Concentrations During Induction and Not HLA-DQA1*05 Carriage is Associated with Anti-Drug Antibody Formation in Patients with Inflammatory Bowel Disease. Gastroenterology 2022. https://doi.org/10.1053/j.gastro.2022.01.009.

117. Colman RJ, Xiong Y, Mizuno T, et al. Antibodies-to-infliximab accelerate clearance while dose intensification reverses immunogenicity and recaptures clinical response in paediatric Crohn's disease. Aliment Pharmacol Ther 2022;55(5): 593–603.

118. van Schaik RHN, Müller DJ, Serretti A, et al. Pharmacogenetics in Psychiatry: An Update on Clinical Usability. Front Pharmacol 2020;11:575540.

119. van der Valk ME, Mangen MJ, Leenders M, et al. Healthcare costs of inflammatory bowel disease have shifted from hospitalisation and surgery towards anti-TNFα therapy: results from the COIN study. Gut 2014;63(1):72–9.

120. Pillai N, Lupatsch JE, Dusheiko M, et al. Evaluating the Cost-Effectiveness of Early Compared with Late or No Biologic Treatment to Manage Crohn's Disease using Real-World Data. J Crohns Colitis 2020;14(4):490–500.

121. Becker C. *Decreasing Drug Costs Through Generics and Biosimilars*. National Conference of State Legislatures. Available at: https://www.ncsl.org/research/health/decreasing-drug-costs-through-biosimilars.aspx#:~:text=For%20a%20biosimilar%20to%20be,prices%20of%20the%20reference%20products. Accessed January 21, 2022.

122. de Groof EJ, Stevens TW, Eshuis EJ, et al. Cost-effectiveness of laparoscopic ileocaecal resection versus infliximab treatment of terminal ileitis in Crohn's disease: the LIR!C Trial. Gut 2019;68(10):1774–80.

123. Bloudek LM, Pandey R, Fazioli K, et al. Optimal treatment sequence for targeted immune modulators for the treatment of moderate to severe ulcerative colitis. J Manag Care Spec Pharm 2021;27(8):1046–55.

124. Siegel CA. Shared decision making in inflammatory bowel disease: helping patients understand the tradeoffs between treatment options. Gut 2012;61(3):459.

125. Schubert S, Picker N, Cavlar T, et al. Inflammatory Bowel Disease Patients' Treatment Preferences Using a Discrete Choice Experiment Technique: The InPuT Study. Adv Ther 2022;39(6):2889–905.

126. Overton PM, Shalet N, Somers F, et al. Patient Preferences for Subcutaneous versus Intravenous Administration of Treatment for Chronic Immune System Disorders: A Systematic Review. Patient Prefer Adherence 2021;15:811–34.

127. Jonaitis L, Marković S, Farkas K, et al. Intravenous versus subcutaneous delivery of biotherapeutics in IBD: an expert's and patient's perspective. BMC Proc 2021;15(17):25.

Safety Summary of Pediatric Inflammatory Bowel Disease Therapies

Xiaoyi Zhang, MD, PhD[a], Joel R. Rosh, MD[b],*

KEYWORDS

- Inflammatory bowel disease • Pediatric • Therapy • Safety

KEY POINTS

- Treatment options for pediatric inflammatory bowel disease (IBD) include aminosalicylates, enteral nutrition, corticosteroids, immunomodulators (thiopurines, methotrexate), biologics, and emerging small molecule agents.
- Thiopurine use increases the risk of rare but serious malignancies including hepatosplenic T-cell lymphoma and Epstein–Barr virus (EBV)-associated lymphoproliferative disorders. This may warrant baseline screening for EBV exposure when considering therapy choice as this risk has not been well-attributed to anti-tumor necrosis factor (TNF) agents and other biologics.
- Approved biologic therapies for pediatric IBD are limited to anti-TNF agents. Baseline infectious screens for tuberculosis and hepatitis B are recommended before initiating therapy. Less common adverse events include infusion reactions, psoriatic-like skin lesions, infections, and other autoimmune-type reactions.
- Newer classes of biologic agents and small molecule inhibitors on the horizon in pediatric IBD care include those targeted against IL-12 and IL-23, leukocyte trafficking via integrin cell adhesion interactions, sphingosine-1-phosphate, and Janus kinase and other tyrosine kinases. Unique risks associated with some of these therapies include metabolic (lipid) derangements, herpes zoster infection, and venous thromboembolic risk, though pediatric data remain limited.

INTRODUCTION

Pediatric patients account for nearly a quarter of those newly diagnosed with inflammatory bowel disease (IBD), and there is increasing global incidence.[1] Although

[a] Pediatric Gastroenterology, Department of Pediatrics, Division of Gastroenterology, Hepatology and Nutrition, Indiana University, 705 Riley Hospital Drive, ROC 4210, Indianapolis, IN 46202, USA; [b] Pediatric Gastroenterology, Division of Pediatric Gastroenterology, Liver Disease, and Nutrition, Cohen Children's Medical Center of New York, 1991 Marcus Avenue, Suite M100, Lake Success, NY 11042, USA
* Corresponding author.
E-mail address: JRosh1@northwell.edu
Twitter: @xtzhang (X.Z.)

Gastroenterol Clin N Am 52 (2023) 535–548
https://doi.org/10.1016/j.gtc.2023.05.007
0889-8553/23/© 2023 Elsevier Inc. All rights reserved.

heterogeneity exists, pediatric patients often face a more aggressive, treatment-refractory disease course with increased disease year burden and associated morbidities.[2] Goals of therapy are to achieve a state of both clinical remission and mucosal healing or so-called deep remission while limiting long-term complications both from ongoing intestinal inflammation and potential secondary adverse events from available therapies. Therapeutic options can include local agents with anti-inflammatory effect via oral or rectal administration, such as aminosalicylates and nonsystemic steroids, as well as methods of systemic immunosuppression with corticosteroids, immunomodulators, biologic drugs, and small molecule agents. Within pediatric care, enteral nutrition is a well-accepted steroid-sparing therapy, especially in Crohn's disease, and is reviewed in detail in this issue. Other treatment strategies lacking substantial clinical data such as combination antibiotics, fecal transplantation, and other investigational therapies will not be reviewed. Novel biologic and small molecule agents with approval in adult IBD and awaiting pediatric studies will be briefly discussed.

Aminosalicylates

Aminosalicylates (mesalamines, sulfasalazine) are locally acting anti-inflammatory agents that inhibit the cyclooxygenase enzymes that mediate prostaglandin production and peroxisome proliferator-activated receptor signaling. Mesalamines are commonly used as first-line maintenance therapy in mild to moderate pediatric ulcerative colitis and provide long-term steroid-free remission in approximately 40% of patients.[3] Sulfasalazine is composed of a 5-aminosalicylic acid (5-ASA) moiety with sulfapyridine carrier, allowing enhanced delivery to the colon. Adverse effects associated with sulfasalazine use, primarily headache and gastrointestinal symptoms and more rarely cytopenias due to inhibited folate metabolism, are most often associated with the sulfapyridine agent and can occur in upward of a third of patients.[4,5] However, its sulfa-compound may provide some benefit toward systemic arthropathies and is the sole salicylate agent available as a liquid preparation. To date, little evidence exists demonstrating clinical superiority or decreased adverse effects among various mesalamine formulations or dosing strategies, if the mesalamine dose is equivalent.[6]

The most common adverse events reported with mesalamine use include worsened symptoms of ulcerative colitis, nausea, and headache.[7] Although worsening gastrointestinal symptoms may be attributable to primary lack of response to therapy or secondary loss of response with disease progression, there exist reports of paradoxical worsening of colitis symptoms, improved by mesalamine drug withdrawal, with several guidelines recommending cessation of mesalamine therapy in the setting of acute severe colitis.[8] Suggested mechanisms include secretory diarrhea driven by alterations in intestinal $Na+/K + ATPase$ and arachidonic acid metabolism.[9,10] In addition, patients with hypersensitivity reactions to aspirin may have cross-reactivity with other salicylate compounds, requiring either desensitization or alternate therapy.[11]

Pancreatitis has been reported in 0.3% to 1.8% of patients on mesalamines with isolated reports in pediatric patients.[6,12] Serious cardiac events, including cardiomyopathy, myocardial infarction, conduction abnormalities, and ventricular dysfunction, are exceedingly rare, with estimated incidences of 0% to 0.3%.[13] 5-ASA-induced myocarditis or pericarditis often presents within the first month of starting therapy, typically with chest pain and accompanying electrocardiogram (EKG) findings, although similar changes have been attributed to extraintestinal manifestations of IBD.[9,14] Cardiac inflammation typically resolves on cessation of 5-ASA therapy but may recur if rechallenged with the same therapy, necessitating definitive drug withdrawal.[15] Nephrotoxicity, manifesting as proteinuria, interstitial nephritis, and even renal failure, has been reported with 5-ASA use, typically occurring within the first year of treatment.[6] Obtaining a baseline serum creatinine in addition to 6 months after therapy and on an annual basis is recommended. Rare case reports of pneumonitis and pneumonia exist, and other reported adverse events include elevated liver enzymes and musculoskeletal complaints (arthralgia, back pain). Impact on male reproductive health, both through sperm function, libido, and erectile dysfunction, has also been reported.[16]

Steroids

Pediatric patients often present with more extensive inflammation and are more likely to require systemic steroids than their adult counterparts. Of note, pediatric patients also have increased risk of steroid-associated complications, most notably growth suppression, but also osteoporosis, glaucoma, and cataracts.[17,18] Corticosteroid therapy increases risk of serious infections to a greater extent than anti-tumor necrosis factor (TNF) therapies in pediatric patients with IBD.[19] Close monitoring is needed for steroid dependency, defined as inability to lower dose or cease therapy within 3 months due to recurrence of symptoms. Such dependency increases the risk of adrenal insufficiency, even following prolonged taper and is associated with low bone density and increased risk of venous thromboembolic events (VTEs).[20,21]

Enteral Nutrition

European guidelines suggest exclusive enteral nutrition as first-line induction therapy in mild to moderate pediatric Crohn's disease and more recent studies of the Crohn's disease exclusion diet provide a less restrictive approach.[22] Although nutritional intervention may be able to both provide symptom and disease control in addition to targeting malnutrition, risks associated with severe dietary restriction in the absence of physician and dietitian-guided support include continued malnutrition, micronutrient deficiencies, and development of avoidant or restrictive food intake practices within a population already at higher risk of these disorders.[23] Additional barriers to successful implementation include expense due to the lack of insurer coverage, formula or diet palatability, social limitations, and fear related to tube feedings.[24]

Methotrexate

Benefits of this immunomodulator include once weekly oral or parenteral administration as well as faster onset of action and potentially lower malignancy risk than thiopurines, but use is often limited by high incidence of gastrointestinal side effects, such as nausea, and requires routine laboratory monitoring for adverse effects including myelosuppression and hepatotoxicity.[25] A recent meta-analysis suggests risk of methotrexate-induced hepatotoxicity and need for therapy discontinuation is increased in adult patients with IBD compared with other inflammatory disorders, although whether disease-specific mechanisms exist which are unclear.[26] There have been rare reports of interstitial pneumonitis, and overall risk of malignancy is unclear, with some suggestion of increased nonmelanoma skin cancers in non-IBD patients.[27] As a known teratogen, its use is strictly contraindicated in pregnancy and recommended for women of child-bearing age with caution and strong consideration of contraception. A washout period of at least 3 months before conception is recommended for women due to the risk of miscarriage and fetal malformation as well as for men due to adverse effects on sperm quality, although the latter recommendation has recently been challenged.[28–30]

Thiopurines

The thiopurines, 6-mercaptopurine (6-MP) and prodrug azathioprine (AZA), are another group of immunomodulators in use since the 1960s as a steroid-sparing agent to maintain disease remission.[31] Identifying therapeutic windows of the active metabolite 6-thioguanine nucleotide is necessary to balance effective immunosuppression while limiting potential adverse events such as cytopenia. Additional monitoring of the downstream thiopurine metabolite 6-methylmercaptopurine may also help prevent hepatotoxicity.[32] Following discovery of specific genetic variants in the thiopurine S-methyltransferase (TPMT) as well as nucleoside diphosphate-linked moiety X-type motif 15, preemptive pharmacogenetic evaluation can identify patients at an increased risk (10–30-fold higher) of severe leukopenia.[33,34] Before initiating therapy, measurement of TPMT enzyme activity or phenotype should be performed. Thiopurine-induced pancreatitis has been reported to occur in approximately 3% of patients, although most cases are mild, improve with drug withdrawal, and may not require permanent drug avoidance.[35]

Thiopurine use is associated with an increased number of general, often mild, viral infections, with more severe presentations associated with specific primary infections such as cytomegalovirus, varicella, and Epstein–Barr virus (EBV). Malignancy risk of thiopurine exposure is most notable for lymphoproliferative disorders. This includes hemophagocytic lymphohistiocytosis in children and adolescents, often associated with a primary EBV infection.[36] The risk of malignancy has been shown to increase after 2 years of thiopurine exposure.[37–39] Absolute risk remains relatively low within pediatric IBD, with a single center cohort detecting an absolute incidence rate of 4.5 per 10,000 patient years of thiopurine use, compared with the expected incidence rate of 0.58.[37] Given the rapid seroconversion of EBV in late adolescence and early adulthood, screening EBV infectious history is recommended before considering thiopurine therapy with suggestion by some guidelines to avoid thiopurine if EBV-naive.[36,38,40,41]

Hepatosplenic T-cell lymphoma, a rare but aggressive malignancy, has been identified in patients with IBD receiving both thiopurine monotherapy and in combination with anti-TNF agents.[39] Additional reports suggest that there is increased risk with thiopurine use alone, with both adult and pediatric cases in males with at least 2 years of thiopurine exposure.[42]

Anti-Tumor Necrosis Factor Therapies

TNF is a pro-inflammatory cytokine which serves as a key driver in many inflammatory and autoimmune disorders. Currently available anti-TNF agents include infliximab, adalimumab, certolizumab, and golimumab, whereas anti-TNF receptor inhibition through etanercept has not been shown to be effective in IBD.

Rates of opportunistic infections have been shown to be approximately twofold higher in adults on anti-TNF therapy, with particular risk for bacteria, fungal, and mycobacterial infections, compared with thiopurine therapy.[43,44] In pediatric patients, rates of serious infections are not increased with anti-TNF use compared with immunomodulator monotherapy and are significantly lower than with corticosteroids.[19,45] Most granulomatous infections associated with anti-TNFs present within the first 6 months, suggesting likely reactivation of a latent infection, predominantly *Mycobacteria tuberculosis*. Within the pediatric population, most of the patients with tuberculosis identified exposures through personal or family foreign-residence, with other risk factors including exposure to a person with untreated active tuberculosis, travel or immunosuppressive therapy.[46] Recommended screening includes the complete evaluation of risk factors, exposures, personal history of Bacillus Calmette-Guerin (BCG) vaccination, and patient symptoms, in addition to screening with tuberculin skin test, with cutoff of 5 mm, interferon-gamma release assay, and/or chest x-ray, with repeat annual screening while on anti-TNF therapy.[47] Rare fungal causes of pneumonia in patients on anti-TNF include Histoplasma, Aspergillus, Coccidioides, and Candida.[48] Patient-specific risk factors including travel or local endemic rates of exposure may warrant preemptive testing.[49] Following anti-TNF treatment, chronic HBV infection may develop into prominent viremia with associated liver injury and more severe complications. Accordingly, anti-hepatitis B surface antibody levels should be performed before the start of anti-TNF therapy to demonstrate adequate seroconversion following immunization and prompt repeated vaccine series administration if low or undetectable.

Potential adverse effects associated with anti-TNF therapy include leukopenia and thrombopenia, with recommendation to monitor at least twice annual complete blood cell counts.[50] Although liver enzyme elevation has been reported with anti-TNF therapy, more serious liver toxicity is rare. Anti-TNFs are contraindicated in patients with later stage heart failure due to worsening function and mortality in early clinical cardiac trials. Within a French database of pediatric patients with IBD, a review of neurologic adverse effects associated with anti-TNF use estimated a total incidence of 1 per 10,000 patient-years.[51]

Acute infusions reactions with infliximab or injection site reactions with adalimumab can range from mild rash or shortness of breath to severe anaphylaxis, often in the setting of antidrug or autoantibody formation.[52] More rarely, delayed manifestations due to hypersensitivity or serum sickness-like reactions can also occur. Therapeutic drug monitoring to assure adequate drug levels and avoid antidrug antibody development can reduce the risk of such reactions.[53] It has recently been noted that carriage of HLA-DQA1*05 allele may be a genetic risk factor for the development of anti-TNF antibodies, even with concomitant immunomodulator use, although a recent pediatric study was unable to confirm this finding.[54–57]

Other adverse autoimmune events associated with anti-TNF blockade include a constellation of inflammatory conditions such as lupus-like syndrome, phospholipid syndrome, vasculitis, multiple sclerosis-like demyelinating disease, peripheral neuropathies, and interstitial lung disease.[58] The induction of new or worsening psoriasiform skin disease has been seen with anti-TNF therapy for both IBD and other autoimmune conditions, often called "paradoxical psoriasis" due to shared inflammatory pathways. The overall prevalence of these anti-TNF-associated psoriatic events is estimated to be less than 3% but a retrospective pediatric study found approximately 11% of patients on anti-TNFs reported skin changes with nearly half being psoriasis.[59] Both in the pediatric cohort and adult reports, most patients with mild to moderate skin manifestations can continue their anti-TNF therapy by "treating through" symptoms and using topical dermatologic agents, often in concert with a dermatologist. Switching to non-anti-TNF therapy is usually reserved for those with poorly controlled underlying disease and/or severe skin eruptions not controlled with topical therapy.[60] A recent retrospective study of 638 pediatric patients found higher rates of both dermatologic symptom resolution and IBD remission following transition to ustekinumab compared with continuing anti-TNF therapy.[60,61]

Adult studies have demonstrated an increased risk of melanoma with anti-TNF use, whereas association with lymphoma risk is conflicting, potentially due to frequent thiopurine exposure.[62–66] Within pediatric patients, the previously cited DEVELOP registry which analyzed 5766 children with IBD over approximately 10 years showed no increased risk of malignancy with infliximab use.[36] Association with hepatosplenic T-cell lymphoma, as discussed earlier, has been primarily associated with thiopurine combination therapy.[42]

Other Anti-Cytokine Agents

Ustekinumab targets the shared interleukin-12 and interleukin-23 p40 subunit, inhibiting the pro-inflammatory cytokine cascade driving activation of T helper type 1 and 17 cells. Since receiving approval for moderate to severe plaque psoriasis, psoriatic arthritis, adult UC, and Crohn's disease, rare adverse events reported include noninfectious pneumonia and acute infusion reactions to the intravenous (IV) but not subcutaneous formulation of ustekinumab.[67,68] Registry data from use in psoriasis have not yet identified any association with malignancies, including nonmelanoma skin cancer, and despite immunosuppressive effects on T-cell activation, there have been no reports of significantly increased risk of intracellular infections or other opportunistic infections.[69–71] Long-term extension IM-UNITI and UNIFI studies in adult Crohn's disease and UC, respectively, have not revealed any new safety concerns.[45,72]

With enhanced understanding of the pathogenic role of Th17 and interleukin (IL)-23 receptor-mediated signaling, supported by animal and human clinical trial data as well as genome-wide association studies, subsequent anti-cytokine antibodies have been developed to specifically target the IL-23 p19 subunit. These therapies include risankizumab, recently approved for use in adult Crohn's disease, with guselkumab, brazikumab, and mirikizumab currently undergoing clinical trials for use in IBD. Phase 3 induction and maintenance withdrawal studies of risankizumab in Crohn's disease have shown excellent tolerance with most common adverse events being headache, nasopharyngitis, and arthralgias and treatment groups showing decreased rates of serious infectious compared with placebo. Overall rates of hepatic events including elevations in liver enzymes and total bilirubin were low (<4%) and did not prompt changes in therapy, though monitoring levels at baseline and repeating within 12 weeks are recommended.[73,74]

Leukocyte Trafficking Therapies

Anti-integrin therapies target leukocyte trafficking into the intestinal tract to limit inflammation. Vedolizumab offers gut-selective targeting of the α4β7-integrin heterodimer, limiting inhibitory effects to interactions with the mucosal addressin-cell adhesion molecule 1 expressed primarily on intestinal endothelium, currently approved in adults for both Crohn's disease (CD) and UC. Owing to gut selectivity, vedolizumab is considered to have among the best safety profiles of available biologic therapies with no increased risk of serious infections, although possible increased risk of mild, non-clostridial enteric infections exist due to its mechanism of action.[75] Currently, long-term safety data are limited, particularly in pediatric patients. A prior single-center study suggested increased risk of postoperative complications in pediatric IBD patients receiving vedolizumab, but additional studies and meta-analyses have not found any significant increase in infections or other postsurgical outcomes.[76]

Janus Kinase Inhibitors

Small molecule inhibition of the Janus kinase (Jak) and signal transducers and activators of transcription pathway, driven by inflammatory cytokines and chemotypes, has resulted in development of several oral agents currently approved or awaiting approval for treatment of ulcerative colitis (UC) in adults, with variable results in CD.[77–79] In addition to oral delivery, these drugs offer rapid onset of action with short half-life and no immunogenicity.[80] The first in-class inhibitor tofacitinib targets primarily Jak1 and Jak3. The selective Jak1 inhibitor upadacitinib was approved in early 2022 for moderate to severe adult UC in adults, with additional inhibitors in development.[81]

Owing to Jak2s role in hematopoiesis, cytopenias are a potential risk of pan-Jak inhibition. In addition to lymphopenia and neutropenia, Jak inhibitors are associated with an increased risk of viral infections. Of these infections, systematic reviews have identified significantly increased risk of herpes zoster infections for patients on tofacitinib (relative risk [RR] 1.72) across all indications.[82] Within IBD, patients of Jak inhibitors have increased risk of infections (RR 1.4), mostly upper respiratory illnesses, although overall rates of herpes zoster were higher than placebo groups, with greatest risk seen in older patients, Asian ethnicity, prior anti-TNF use, and higher dose (10 mg vs 5 mg twice daily).[83,84] Within the pediatric population, rates of primary varicella infection have greatly declined since the 1995 introduction of the two-dose varicella-zoster vaccine.[85] However, inadequate immunization status whether due to age of diagnosis, seroconversion, or other factors remains a concern.

After FDA approval, additional studies primarily in rheumatoid arthritis showed increased risk of major adverse cardiovascular events (MACE) and venous thromboembolism (VTE) in older adults over 50 years of age with at least one cardiovascular risk factor, prompting recommendations to limit use to patients refractory to anti-TNF therapy and attempting to de-escalate dose from 10 mg twice daily if possible. Larger pooled analyses of MACEs in patients treated with Jak inhibitors have not shown a significantly increased risk compared with placebo-controls.[82] However, post-marketing safety trials of tofacitinib in rheumatoid arthritis, revealing increased rates of pulmonary embolism and death, have since limited use in rheumatoid arthritis (RA) to lower 5 mg twice daily dosing. Although total incidents within UC patients remain low and essentially limited to patients over age 50 years with at least one pre-existing risk factor, VTE risk remains a concern, particularly considering additive risk from inflammatory bowel disease activity.[86,87] In addition to increased risk with intestinal inflammation, additional VTE risk factors for patients with IBD include in-dwelling central venous catheter, personal or family history of thromboembolic events, tobacco use, postoperative status, and potentially estrogen-containing contraceptives.[87,88] As in adult patients, pediatric use is currently limited to moderate to severe colitis refractory to anti-TNF therapy with recommendation to attempt to achieve the lowest effective dose and shortest duration needed.

Post-hoc analysis of UC Jak inhibitor trials identified elevated total, low density, and high-density cholesterol levels, typically dose-dependent and reversible, with peak following 8 weeks of therapy and stable through over 1 year follow-up, without associated increased risk of MACEs.[89] Clinical trials also reported elevations of serum creatinine, liver enzymes, and creatinine kinase, without associated liver failure or rhabdomyolysis.[90,91] Although a few patients discontinued therapy due to creatinine kinase and serum creatinine elevations, no patients met discontinuation criteria based on liver function tests.[90] Phase 3 trials of tofacitinib for pediatric patients with juvenile idiopathic arthritis and upadacitinib for atopic dermatitis revealed no new safety concerns compared with adult studies with similar rates of adverse events and serious adverse events across all treatment groups and no reported MACE or thrombotic events.[92,93] Within its use in rheumatoid arthritis, tofacitinib has been associated with increased risk of lung cancer compared with anti-TNF therapy.[94,95] However, this effect has not been seen in a meta-analysis of Jaki use across immune-mediated disorders nor within IBD alone.[82,90]

Sphingosine-1-Phosphate Receptor Modulators

The oral sphingosine-1-phosphate receptor modulator ozanimod prevents lymph node egress of activated T cells and therefore their migration to tissue sites of inflammation. Ozanimod is approved for use in adult UC with pediatric trials ongoing.

Etrasimod has a similar mechanism of action with completion of phase 3 adult studies demonstrating effective induction and maintenance of remission in moderate to severe UC.[96] Common adverse events reported in early S1PR trials include anemia, nasopharyngitis, and headache during induction, with increased elevated liver enzymes and headache in the maintenance phase. Serious associated risks include macular edema, increased in patients with uveitis or diabetes mellitus, and cardiac conduction abnormalities, notably sinus bradycardia and atrioventricular conduction delays, warranting screening EKG before use.[97] Given these risks, use in patients with significant cardiovascular disease or arrhythmias such as Mobitz type II or higher heart blocks is contraindicated.

SUMMARY

Pediatric therapies for inflammatory bowel disease include locally active agents, aminosalicylates and enteral steroids, as well as systemic corticosteroids, nutritional therapy, immunomodulators methotrexate and AZA or 6-MP, and anti-TNF biologics. Additional therapies awaiting approval for pediatric use and other agents in development include biologic agents targeting integrin-mediated leukocyte trafficking, cytokines IL-12 and IL-23, and inhibitors of sphingosine-1-phosphate-mediated leukocyte migration and tyrosine kinase signaling pathways. Potential toxicities from these therapies can include effects on blood cell counts, renal, and liver function with less common adverse events reported, specific to individual agents, which warrant routine clinical and laboratory monitoring. Systemic immunosuppression carries increased infection risk, with recommended universal screening for tuberculosis and hepatitis B before anti-TNF therapy initiation. Rare but serious risks of malignancy have been reported with thiopurine use.

CLINICS CARE POINTS

- For patients on aminosalicylates, monitoring should include assessment of new clinical symptoms at each visit, and annual laboratory monitoring of renal and liver function. Symptoms of pancreatitis, pneumonia, or cardiac disease should warrant focused laboratory and diagnostic studies due to the risk of rare adverse events.

- To limit adverse effects of high-dose, prolonged steroid exposure, consider limiting to 40 mg single daily dose, closely assessing initial clinical symptoms during and immediately following dose taper, and considering additional screens for low bone mineral density and adrenal suppression if prolonged course is needed. Prophylaxis against venous thromboembolic events should be considered in the acute setting in the presence of other risk factors.

- Enteral nutrition can be an effective therapy alone or in conjunction with other therapies. Close monitoring with dietician support is needed to ensure increased energy requirements are met in the setting of malnutrition and active inflammation. Avoidant and restrictive food intake behaviors often develop in patients with inflammatory bowel disease and should be regularly assessed.

- The use of methotrexate should include initial and routine complete blood cell counts, renal and liver function tests, daily folate supplementation, and counseling on contraceptive care for all postpubertal females.

- Assessing thiopurine S-methyltransferase (TPMT) activity level, preferred over genetic evaluation of TPMT, and nucleoside diphosphate-linked moiety X-type motif 15 variants should be performed before starting thiopurine treatment to identify populations at an increased risk of severe leukopenia. The evaluation of Epstein–Barr virus serology may be considered due to risk of severe lymphoproliferative disorders with primary infections. On therapy start, routine monitoring should include serial complete blood cell counts and liver function tests, with additional evaluation if clinical symptoms suggestive of pancreatitis or cholestasis occur. Health maintenance should include routine dermatologic surveillance and routine sun exposure prevention.

- Anti-tumor necrosis factor agents increase risk of infections, primarily driven by intracellular pathogens, and warrant universal screening for tuberculosis and hepatitis B infection before starting therapy, with consideration of other intracellular or opportunistic infections, pending individual risk factors. Potential adverse events include infusion reactions, drug-induced psoriasis, and autoimmune reactions which can range in severity.

- Additional biologic and other novel therapies are not currently approved in pediatrics, with use limited as second- or third-line therapies. Anti-cytokine therapy against IL-12/IL-23 and gut-directed anti-integrin therapy both have excellent safety profiles with limited reports of adverse events in adults.

- Small molecule inhibitors targeting sphingosine-1-phosphate and tyrosine kinase pathways have been approved for use in adult UC; however, pediatric data are currently limited.

DISCLOSURE

X. Zhang Consultant: Janssen. J.R. Rosh: Grant/Research Funding: AbbVie, United States, Janssen, United States; Consultant/Advisory Board: AbbVie, BMS, Janssen, Lilly, Pfizer.

REFERENCES

1. Kuenzig ME, Fung SG, Marderfeld L, et al. Twenty-first Century Trends in the Global Epidemiology of Pediatric-Onset Inflammatory Bowel Disease: Systematic Review. Gastroenterology 2022;162(4):1147–59.
2. Nasiri S, Kuenzig ME, Benchimol EI. Long-term outcomes of pediatric inflammatory bowel disease. Semin Pediatr Surg 2017;26(6):398–404.
3. Hyams JS, Davis Thomas S, Gotman N, et al. Clinical and biological predictors of response to standardised paediatric colitis therapy (PROTECT): a multicentre inception cohort study. Lancet 2019;393(10182):1708–20.
4. Haagen Nielsen O, Bondesen S. Kinetics of 5-aminosalicylic acid after jejunal instillation in man. Br J Clin Pharmacol 1983;16(6):738–40.
5. Selhub J, Dhar GJ, Rosenberg IH. Inhibition of folate enzymes by sulfasalazine. J Clin Invest 1978;61(1):221–4.
6. Sehgal P, Colombel JF, Aboubakr A, et al. Systematic review: safety of mesalazine in ulcerative colitis. Aliment Pharmacol Ther 2018;47(12):1597–609.
7. Sandborn WJ, Regula J, Feagan BG, et al. Delayed-release oral mesalamine 4.8 g/day (800-mg tablet) is effective for patients with moderately active ulcerative colitis. Gastroenterology 2009;137(6):1934–43.
8. Turner D, Ruemmele FM, Orlanski-Meyer E, et al. Management of Paediatric Ulcerative Colitis, Part 2: Acute Severe Colitis-An Evidence-based Consensus Guideline From the European Crohn's and Colitis Organization and the European Society of Paediatric Gastroenterology, Hepatology and Nutrition. J Pediatr Gastroenterol Nutr 2018;67(2):292–310.
9. Scheurlen C, Allgayer H, Kruis W, et al. Effect of olsalazine and mesalazine on human ileal and colonic (Na+ + K+)-ATPase. A possible diarrhogenic factor? Clin Investig 1993;71(4):286–9.
10. Fine KD, Sarles HE, Cryer B. Diarrhea associated with mesalamine in a patient with chronic nongranulomatous enterocolitis. N Engl J Med 1998;338(13):923–5.

11. Heath JL, Heath RD, Tamboli C, et al. Mesalamine desensitization in a patient with treatment refractory ulcerative colitis and aspirin and nonsteroidal anti-inflammatory drug hypersensitivity. Ann Allergy Asthma Immunol 2017;118(4): 518–20.

12. Keljo DJ, Sugerman KS. Pancreatitis in patients with inflammatory bowel disease. J Pediatr Gastroenterol Nutr 1997;25(1):108–12.

13. Sandborn WJ, Korzenik J, Lashner B, et al. Once-daily dosing of delayed-release oral mesalamine (400-mg tablet) is as effective as twice-daily dosing for maintenance of remission of ulcerative colitis. Gastroenterology 2010;138(4):1286–96.

14. Cesa K, Cunningham C, Harris T, et al. A Review of Extraintestinal Manifestations & Medication-Induced Myocarditis and Pericarditis in Pediatric Inflammatory Bowel Disease. Cureus 2022;14(6):e26366.

15. Brown G. 5-Aminosalicylic Acid-Associated Myocarditis and Pericarditis: A Narrative Review. Can J Hosp Pharm 2016;69(6):466–72.

16. Shin T, Kobori Y, Suzuki K, et al. Inflammatory bowel disease in subfertile men and the effect of mesalazine on fertility. Syst Biol Reprod Med 2014;60(6):373–6.

17. Van Limbergen J, Russell RK, Drummond HE, et al. Definition of phenotypic characteristics of childhood-onset inflammatory bowel disease. Gastroenterology 2008;135(4):1114–22.

18. Uchida K, Araki T, Toiyama Y, et al. Preoperative steroid-related complications in Japanese pediatric patients with ulcerative colitis. Dis Colon Rectum 2006; 49(1):74–9.

19. Dulai PS, Thompson KD, Blunt HB, et al. Risks of serious infection or lymphoma with anti-tumor necrosis factor therapy for pediatric inflammatory bowel disease: a systematic review. Clin Gastroenterol Hepatol 2014;12(9):1443–51.

20. Sidoroff M, Kolho K-L. Screening for adrenal suppression in children with inflammatory bowel disease discontinuing glucocorticoid therapy. BMC Gastroenterol 2014;14:51.

21. Rozes S, Guilmin-Crepon S, Alison M, et al. Bone health in pediatric patients with Crohn disease. J Pediatr Gastroenterol Nutr 2021;73(2):231–5.

22. Levine A, Wine E, Assa A, et al. Crohn's disease exclusion diet plus partial enteral nutrition induces sustained remission in a randomized controlled trial. Gastroenterology 2019;157(2):440–50.

23. Yelencich E, Truong E, Widaman AM, et al. Avoidant restrictive food intake disorder prevalent among patients with inflammatory bowel disease. Clin Gastroenterol Hepatol 2022;20(6):1282–9.

24. Green N, Miller T, Suskind D, et al. A review of dietary therapy for IBD and a vision for the future. Nutrients 2019;(5):11.

25. Herfarth HH. Methotrexate for Inflammatory Bowel Diseases - New Developments. Dig Dis 2016;34(1–2):140–6.

26. Wang Y, Li Y, Liu Y, et al. Patients With IBD Receiving Methotrexate Are at Higher Risk of Liver Injury Compared With Patients With Non-IBD Diseases: A Meta-Analysis and Systematic Review. Front Med 2021;8:774824.

27. Ridker PM, Everett BM, Pradhan A, et al. Low-Dose Methotrexate for the Prevention of Atherosclerotic Events. N Engl J Med 2019;380(8):752–62.

28. Cao RH, Grimm MC. Pregnancy and medications in inflammatory bowel disease. Obstet Med 2021;14(1):4–11.

29. Dawson AL, Riehle-Colarusso T, Reefhuis J, et al. National Birth Defects Prevention Study. Maternal exposure to methotrexate and birth defects: a population-based study. Am J Med Genet 2014;164A(9):2212–6.

30. Grosen A, Bellaguarda E, Nersting J, et al. Low-dose Methotrexate Therapy Does Not Affect Semen Parameters and Sperm DNA. Inflamm Bowel Dis 2022;28(7): 1012–8.

31. Kapur S, Hanauer SB. The evolving role of thiopurines in inflammatory bowel disease. Curr Treat Options Gastroenterol 2019;17(3):420–33.

32. González-Lama Y, Gisbert JP. Monitoring thiopurine metabolites in inflammatory bowel disease. Frontline Gastroenterol 2016;7(4):301–7.

33. Walker GJ, Harrison JW, Heap GA, et al. Association of Genetic Variants in NUDT15 With Thiopurine-Induced Myelosuppression in Patients With Inflammatory Bowel Disease. JAMA 2019;321(8):773–85.

34. Roberts RL, Barclay ML. Update on thiopurine pharmacogenetics in inflammatory bowel disease. Pharmacogenomics 2015;16(8):891–903.

35. Ledder OD, Lemberg DA, Ooi CY, et al. Are thiopurines always contraindicated after thiopurine-induced pancreatitis in inflammatory bowel disease? J Pediatr Gastroenterol Nutr 2013;57(5):583–6.

36. Hyams JS, Dubinsky MC, Baldassano RN, et al. Infliximab is not associated with increased risk of malignancy or hemophagocytic lymphohistiocytosis in pediatric patients with inflammatory bowel disease. Gastroenterology 2017;152(8): 1901–14.

37. Ashworth LA, Billett A, Mitchell P, et al. Lymphoma risk in children and young adults with inflammatory bowel disease: analysis of a large single-center cohort. Inflamm Bowel Dis 2012;18(5):838–43.

38. Beaugerie L, Brousse N, Bouvier AM, et al. Lymphoproliferative disorders in patients receiving thiopurines for inflammatory bowel disease: a prospective observational cohort study. Lancet 2009;374(9701):1617–25.

39. Kotlyar DS, Lewis JD, Beaugerie L, et al. Risk of lymphoma in patients with inflammatory bowel disease treated with azathioprine and 6-mercaptopurine: a meta-analysis. Clin Gastroenterol Hepatol 2015;13(5):847–58.

40. Linton MS, Kroeker K, Fedorak D, et al. Prevalence of Epstein-Barr Virus in a population of patients with inflammatory bowel disease: a prospective cohort study. Aliment Pharmacol Ther 2013;38(10):1248–54.

41. Annese V, Beaugerie L, Egan L, et al. European Evidence-based Consensus: Inflammatory Bowel Disease and Malignancies. J Crohns Colitis 2015;9(11): 945–65.

42. Kotlyar DS, Osterman MT, Diamond RH, et al. A systematic review of factors that contribute to hepatosplenic T-cell lymphoma in patients with inflammatory bowel disease. Clin Gastroenterol Hepatol 2011;9(1):36–41.

43. Ford AC, Peyrin-Biroulet L. Opportunistic infections with anti-tumor necrosis factor-α therapy in inflammatory bowel disease: meta-analysis of randomized controlled trials. Am J Gastroenterol 2013;108(8):1268–76.

44. Kirchgesner J, Lemaitre M, Carrat F, et al. Risk of serious and opportunistic infections associated with treatment of inflammatory bowel diseases. Gastroenterology 2018;155(2):337–46.

45. Sandborn WJ, Rebuck R, Wang Y, et al. Five-Year Efficacy and Safety of Ustekinumab Treatment in Crohn's Disease: The IM-UNITI Trial. Clin Gastroenterol Hepatol 2022;20(3):578–90.

46. Winston CA, Menzies HJ. Pediatric and adolescent tuberculosis in the United States, 2008-2010. Pediatrics 2012;130(6):e1425–32.

47. Starke JR, Committee. On Infectious Diseases. Interferon-γ release assays for diagnosis of tuberculosis infection and disease in children. Pediatrics 2014; 134(6):e1763–73.

48. Wallis RS, Broder MS, Wong JY, et al. Granulomatous infectious diseases associated with tumor necrosis factor antagonists. Clin Infect Dis 2004;38(9):1261–5.

49. Ordonez ME, Farraye FA, Di Palma JA. Endemic fungal infections in inflammatory bowel disease associated with anti-TNF antibody therapy. Inflamm Bowel Dis 2013;19(11):2490–500.

50. Shivaji UN, Sharratt CL, Thomas T, et al. Review article: managing the adverse events caused by anti-TNF therapy in inflammatory bowel disease. Aliment Pharmacol Ther 2019;49(6):664–80.

51. Bertrand V, Massy N, Pigneur B, et al. Neurological Adverse Effects Associated With Anti-tumor Necrosis Factor Alpha Antibodies in Pediatric Inflammatory Bowel Diseases. J Pediatr Gastroenterol Nutr 2020;70(6):841–8.

52. Friesen CA, Calabro C, Christenson K, et al. Safety of infliximab treatment in pediatric patients with inflammatory bowel disease. J Pediatr Gastroenterol Nutr 2004;39(3):265–9.

53. Papamichael K, Chachu KA, Vajravelu RK, et al. Improved Long-term Outcomes of Patients With Inflammatory Bowel Disease Receiving Proactive Compared With Reactive Monitoring of Serum Concentrations of Infliximab. Clin Gastroenterol Hepatol 2017;15(10):1580–8.

54. Syversen SW, Jørgensen KK, Goll GL, et al. Effect of Therapeutic Drug Monitoring vs Standard Therapy During Maintenance Infliximab Therapy on Disease Control in Patients With Immune-Mediated Inflammatory Diseases: A Randomized Clinical Trial. JAMA 2021;326(23):2375–84.

55. Sazonovs A, Kennedy NA, Moutsianas L, et al. HLA-DQA1*05 Carriage Associated With Development of Anti-Drug Antibodies to Infliximab and Adalimumab in Patients With Crohn's Disease. Gastroenterology 2020;158(1):189–99.

56. Choi B, Sey M, Ponich T, et al. Decreased infliximab concentrations in patients with inflammatory bowel disease who carry a variable number tandem repeat polymorphism in the neonatal fc receptor or variant HLADQA1*05G>A genotype. Inflamm Bowel Dis 2023;29(3):437–43.

57. Colman RJ, Xiong Y, Mizuno T, et al. Antibodies-to-infliximab accelerate clearance while dose intensification reverses immunogenicity and recaptures clinical response in paediatric Crohn's disease. Aliment Pharmacol Ther 2022;55(5):593–603.

58. Prinz JC. Autoimmune-like syndromes during TNF blockade: does infection have a role? Nat Rev Rheumatol 2011;7(7):429–34.

59. Sridhar S, Maltz RM, Boyle B, et al. Dermatological Manifestations in Pediatric Patients with Inflammatory Bowel Diseases on Anti-TNF Therapy. Inflamm Bowel Dis 2018;24(9):2086–92.

60. Li SJ, Perez-Chada LM, Merola JF. TNF Inhibitor-Induced Psoriasis: Proposed Algorithm for Treatment and Management. J Psoriasis Psoriatic Arthritis 2019;4(2):70–80.

61. Dolinger MT, Rolfes P, Spencer E, et al. Outcomes of Children with Inflammatory Bowel Disease who Develop Anti-tumour Necrosis Factor-induced Skin Reactions. J Crohns Colitis 2022;16(9):1420–7.

62. Osterman MT, Sandborn WJ, Colombel J-F, et al. Increased risk of malignancy with adalimumab combination therapy, compared with monotherapy, for Crohn's disease. Gastroenterology 2014;146(4):941–9.

63. Long MD, Martin CF, Pipkin CA, et al. Risk of melanoma and nonmelanoma skin cancer among patients with inflammatory bowel disease. Gastroenterology 2012;143(2):390–9.

64. Nyboe Andersen N, Pasternak B, Basit S, et al. Association between tumor necrosis factor-α antagonists and risk of cancer in patients with inflammatory bowel disease. JAMA 2014;311(23):2406–13.

65. Lichtenstein GR, Feagan BG, Cohen RD, et al. Drug therapies and the risk of malignancy in Crohn's disease: results from the TREATTM Registry. Am J Gastroenterol 2014;109(2):212–23.

66. Lemaitre M, Kirchgesner J, Rudnichi A, et al. Association between use of thiopurines or tumor necrosis factor antagonists alone or in combination and risk of lymphoma in patients with inflammatory bowel disease. JAMA 2017;318(17):1679–86.

67. Mitchel EB, Paul A, El-Ali A, et al. Drug-induced Lung Disease Associated With Ustekinumab in a Pediatric Patient With Crohn Disease. J Pediatr Gastroenterol Nutr 2020;71(5):e143–5.

68. Spencer EA, Kinnucan J, Wang J, et al. Real-World Experience With Acute Infusion Reactions to Ustekinumab at 2 Large Tertiary Care Centers. Crohns Colitis 360 2020;2(2). https://doi.org/10.1093/crocol/otaa022.

69. Kalb RE, Fiorentino DF, Lebwohl MG, et al. Risk of serious infection with biologic and systemic treatment of psoriasis: results from the psoriasis longitudinal assessment and registry (PSOLAR). JAMA Dermatol 2015;151(9):961–9.

70. Langley RG, Lebwohl M, Krueger GG, et al. Long term efficacy and safety of ustekinumab, with and without dosing adjustment, in patients with moderate-to-severe psoriasis: results from the PHOENIX 2 study through 5 years of follow-up. Br J Dermatol 2015;172(5):1371–83.

71. Fiorentino D, Ho V, Lebwohl MG, et al. Risk of malignancy with systemic psoriasis treatment in the Psoriasis Longitudinal Assessment Registry. J Am Acad Dermatol 2017;77(5):845–54.

72. Abreu MT, Rowbotham DS, Danese S, et al. Efficacy and Safety of Maintenance Ustekinumab for Ulcerative Colitis Through 3 Years: UNIFI Long-term Extension. J Crohns Colitis 2022;16(8):1222–34.

73. D'Haens G, Panaccione R, Baert F, et al. Risankizumab as induction therapy for Crohn's disease: results from the phase 3 ADVANCE and MOTIVATE induction trials. Lancet 2022;399(10340):2015–30.

74. Ferrante M, Panaccione R, Baert F, et al. Risankizumab as maintenance therapy for moderately to severely active Crohn's disease: results from the multicentre, randomised, double-blind, placebo-controlled, withdrawal phase 3 FORTIFY maintenance trial. Lancet 2022;399(10340):2031–46.

75. Colombel J-F, Sands BE, Rutgeerts P, et al. The safety of vedolizumab for ulcerative colitis and Crohn's disease. Gut 2017;66(5):839–51.

76. Yung DE, Horesh N, Lightner AL, et al. Systematic Review and Meta-analysis: Vedolizumab and Postoperative Complications in Inflammatory Bowel Disease. Inflamm Bowel Dis 2018;24(11):2327–38.

77. Villarino AV, Kanno Y, O'Shea JJ. Mechanisms and consequences of Jak-STAT signaling in the immune system. Nat Immunol 2017;18(4):374–84.

78. Salas A, Hernandez-Rocha C, Duijvestein M, et al. JAK-STAT pathway targeting for the treatment of inflammatory bowel disease. Nat Rev Gastroenterol Hepatol 2020;17(6):323–37.

79. Panés J, Sandborn WJ, Schreiber S, et al. Tofacitinib for induction and maintenance therapy of Crohn's disease: results of two phase IIb randomised placebo-controlled trials. Gut 2017;66(6):1049–59.

80. Hanauer S, Panaccione R, Danese S, et al. Tofacitinib induction therapy reduces symptoms within 3 days for patients with ulcerative colitis. Clin Gastroenterol Hepatol 2019;17(1):139–47.

81. Grossberg LB, Papamichael K, Cheifetz AS. Review article: emerging drug therapies in inflammatory bowel disease. Aliment Pharmacol Ther 2022;55(7):789–804.

82. Olivera PA, Lasa JS, Bonovas S, et al. Safety of Janus Kinase Inhibitors in Patients With Inflammatory Bowel Diseases or Other Immune-mediated Diseases: A Systematic Review and Meta-Analysis. Gastroenterology 2020;158(6):1554–73.

83. Ma C, Lee JK, Mitra AR, et al. Systematic review with meta-analysis: efficacy and safety of oral Janus kinase inhibitors for inflammatory bowel disease. Aliment Pharmacol Ther 2019;50(1):5–23.

84. Winthrop KL, Melmed GY, Vermeire S, et al. Herpes zoster infection in patients with ulcerative colitis receiving tofacitinib. Inflamm Bowel Dis 2018;24(10):2258–65.

85. Marin M, Zhang JX, Seward JF. Near elimination of varicella deaths in the US after implementation of the vaccination program. Pediatrics 2011;128(2):214–20.

86. Sandborn WJ, Panés J, Sands BE, et al. Venous thromboembolic events in the tofacitinib ulcerative colitis clinical development programme. Aliment Pharmacol Ther 2019;50(10):1068–76.

87. Cheng K, Faye AS. Venous thromboembolism in inflammatory bowel disease. World J Gastroenterol 2020;26(12):1231–41.

88. Limdi JK, Farraye J, Cannon R, et al. Contraception, venous thromboembolism, and inflammatory bowel disease: what clinicians (and patients) should know. Inflamm Bowel Dis 2019;25(10):1603–12.

89. Sands BE, Taub PR, Armuzzi A, et al. Tofacitinib treatment is associated with modest and reversible increases in serum lipids in patients with ulcerative colitis. Clin Gastroenterol Hepatol 2020;18(1):123–32.

90. Sandborn WJ, Panés J, D'Haens GR, et al. Safety of tofacitinib for treatment of ulcerative colitis, based on 4.4 years of data from global clinical trials. Clin Gastroenterol Hepatol 2019;17(8):1541–50.

91. Valenzuela F, Korman NJ, Bissonnette R, et al. Tofacitinib in patients with moderate-to-severe chronic plaque psoriasis: long-term safety and efficacy in an open-label extension study. Br J Dermatol 2018;179(4):853–62.

92. Ruperto N, Brunner HI, Synoverska O, et al. Tofacitinib in juvenile idiopathic arthritis: a double-blind, placebo-controlled, withdrawal phase 3 randomised trial. Lancet 2021;398(10315):1984–96.

93. Katoh N, Ohya Y, Murota H, et al. A phase 3 randomized, multicenter, double-blind study to evaluate the safety of upadacitinib in combination with topical corticosteroids in adolescent and adult patients with moderate-to-severe atopic dermatitis in Japan (Rising Up): An interim 24-week analysis. JAAD International 2022;6:27–36.

94. Curtis JR, Lee EB, Kaplan IV, et al. Tofacitinib, an oral Janus kinase inhibitor: analysis of malignancies across the rheumatoid arthritis clinical development programme. Ann Rheum Dis 2016;75(5):831–41.

95. Curtis JR, Yamaoka K, Chen Y-H, et al. Malignancy risk with tofacitinib versus TNF inhibitors in rheumatoid arthritis: results from the open-label, randomised controlled ORAL Surveillance trial. Ann Rheum Dis 2023;82(3):331–43.

96. Sandborn WJ, Vermeire S, Peyrin-Biroulet L, et al. Etrasimod as induction and maintenance therapy for ulcerative colitis (ELEVATE): two randomised, double-blind, placebo-controlled, phase 3 studies. Lancet 2023. https://doi.org/10.1016/S0140-6736(23)00061-2.

97. Sandborn WJ, Feagan BG, D'Haens G, et al. Ozanimod as induction and maintenance therapy for ulcerative colitis. N Engl J Med 2021;385(14):1280–91.

The Role of Therapeutic Drug Monitoring in Children

Alexander Nasr, MD[a], Phillip Minar, MD, MS[a,b],*

KEYWORDS

- Proactive Drug monitoring • Drug concentrations • Pharmacokinetics
- Inflammatory bowel disease

KEY POINTS

- Biologics are a mainstay of therapy in pediatric IBD, first-line for moderate-severe Crohn's disease and second line for moderate-severe ulcerative colitis.
- Children with IBD on biologics have been found to have significantly different pharmacokinetics than adults, especially the small (<30 kg), young (<10 years) child.
- Multiple patient-specific factors (biomarkers) have been found to alter the clearance of biologics further highlighting the need for predictive tools to allow for individualized dosing to achieve therapeutic target concentrations.
- Proactive therapeutic drug monitoring with a drug-tolerant assay is a key to preemptively check for rapid drug clearance and early immunogenicity.

BACKGROUND

Inflammatory bowel disease (IBD), which includes Crohn's disease (CD) and ulcerative colitis (UC), affects over three million people in the United States, with up to a quarter of new diagnoses occurring in childhood.[1] While pediatric and adult-onset IBD share similar therapeutic goals, management of pediatric IBD presents distinct challenges. Specifically, the additional hurdles include growth delays in both pre- and post-pubertal children, often a more extensive inflammatory burden (children more commonly present with ileocolonic CD and UC-pancolitis), reduced access to novel therapeutics and unique drug (biologic) pharmacokinetics (PK), especially in the young, early-onset patients with IBD (<10 year old and <30 kg).[2–4] Given these unique challenges, there is an urgency to optimize medical management to rapidly induce and maintain clinical remission, prevent growth delays, maximize the quality of life, and minimize long-term complications by targeting mucosal healing.[5]

[a] Division of Pediatric Gastroenterology, Hepatology & Nutrition, Cincinnati Children's Hospital Medical Center, MLC 2010, 3333 Burnet Avenue, Cincinnati, OH 45229, USA; [b] Department of Pediatrics, University of Cincinnati School of Medicine, Cincinnati, OH, USA
* Corresponding author.
E-mail address: phillip.minar@cchmc.org

Gastroenterol Clin N Am 52 (2023) 549–563
https://doi.org/10.1016/j.gtc.2023.05.002
0889-8553/23/© 2023 Elsevier Inc. All rights reserved.

The recognition of this limited "window of opportunity" to prevent IBD-related complications has resulted in an emphasis on early diagnosis, frequent use of surrogate biomarkers, judicious use of repeat abdominal imaging or endoscopy and more prompt use of top-down therapy. Hence, the management of pediatric IBD has quickly shifted from simply controlling gastrointestinal symptoms to implementing a treat-to-target approach with a primary focus on proactive therapeutic adjustments targeting endoscopic healing to prevent IBD-related complications.[5] Other than a subgroup of patients with UC responding to a 5-aminosalicylates, past studies have shown that use of immunomodulators (IMM) and corticosteroids (CS) result in subpar rates of endoscopic healing[6] and less than ideal rates of clinical remission.[7] With favorable safety and effectiveness data from the first clinical trials and real-world use, biologics have become the mainstay of moderate-severe IBD.[8,9]

While initial PK studies with biologics may have suggested similar PK parameters between children and adults, in real-world practice many patients on standard (as-labeled) dosing regimens require frequent dose intensification to achieve clinical, endoscopic or transmural remission.[4,10–14] Nonresponse to a biologic may be multifactorial, however, often there is a direct correlation between a low drug concentration or presence of neutralizing anti-drug antibodies (ADA) and more severe disease activity.[2,15,16] Now, with the widespread adoption of therapeutic drug monitoring (TDM) in pediatric IBD management, one clinical trial and severe real-world studies have shown improved outcomes when specific drug concentrations are achieved and ADAs are minimized.[4,17,18] Despite these favorable studies of use of proactive TDM in children, the American Gastroenterological Association (AGA) published guidelines support the use of reactive TDM in adults with IBD, with scarce guidance for those caring for children.[19] In this review, our primary objective is to highlight the importance of both reactive and proactive TDM in guiding biologic dose and frequency for children with IBD.

CURRENT EVIDENCE
Thiopurine Therapeutic Drug Monitoring Kicks off Treating to a Target

Use of TDM to titrate exposure to antibiotics and other immunosuppressive therapies is well established and has been associated with improved outcomes.[20,21] It was not until 2000, that Dubinsky and colleagues reported that 6-mercaptopurine metabolite concentrations (6-TG and 6-MMP) and thiopurine S-methyltransferase (TPMT) genotyping was key to achieving improved IBD outcomes and minimizing drug toxicity.[22] While use of 6-mercaptopurine in children has declined with preferential use of the anti-TNF biologics as the first-line therapy for moderate to severe CD, this initial study of TDM use in IBD care provided the framework for which optimized biologic dosing to achieve a therapeutic target is based.

Use of Therapeutic Drug Monitoring with Biologics

The Food and Drug Administration (FDA) first approved infliximab and adalimumab for pediatric (≥6 years of age) use in 2006 and 2012, respectively. In contrast, the more novel biologics, vedolizumab (anti-integrin), ustekinumab (anti-IL12/23), and risankizumab (anti-IL23) are only approved for adult-onset IBD (≥18 year old) with any use of these biologics in children considered "off-label." As the anti-TNF biologics, infliximab, and adalimumab, are the only monoclonal antibodies currently FDA-approved for use in children, this review will primarily focus on the use of anti-TNF TDM with a shorter review of the off-label dosing guidelines for the other biologics.

Understanding the Type of Assay is Key to Interpreting Therapeutic Drug Monitoring

As the development of ADA (immunogenicity) is known to increase drug clearance and diminish response,[2,10] the key to assessing drug effectiveness in clinical practice requires the use of a drug detection assay that can quantify both drug and ADA (a drug-tolerant assay) in the same sample. Interpretation of early TDM studies was more limited as the first commercially available assays for biologic concentrations were only able to detect ADAs when the drug was undetectable (a drug-sensitive assay). Therefore, to interpret TDM, the clinician must first be aware of the type of TDM assay (whether drug-tolerant or drug-sensitive) used, whether the drug concentration measured includes free (unbound) or total (bound and unbound) drug concentration and whether the ADA detected are neutralizing or non-neutralizing antibodies. Often, these complexities of TDM interpretation may be minimized by repeated use (familiarity) of the same assay for a single patient or the entire practice.

While there is an ongoing debate about the influence of "low-level" anti-drug antibodies on drug clearance, Colman and colleagues showed that patients with the lowest detectable ADA (23 ng/mL) to infliximab had an impact on drug clearance.[2]

As routine use and insurance coverage of TDM expands, there are now more commercially available assays. These include the enzyme-linked immunosorbent assay (ELISA), the homogenous mobility shift assay (HMSA), the electrochemiluminescence immunoassay (ECLIA), and a cell-based bioassay to quantify drug inhibition. Additional studies are still needed to directly compare all commercially available assays as those that have been performed have shown variable correlations which is beyond the scope of this review.[23,24]

Critical Benefits from Reactive Therapeutic Drug Monitoring

Gastroenterologists are well versed in assessing TPMT activity or genotyping to inform dose selection for patients with IBD starting 6-mercaptopurine or azathioprine. While TPMT genotyping is used for initial dose selection, clinicians often relied on "reactive" metabolite testing when the patient presented with an acute increase in gastrointestinal symptoms, elevation of surrogate blood or stool biomarkers, concern for drug toxicity or there was evidence of gut inflammation by colonoscopy. In general, reactive TDM in these cases was an opportunity to assess drug adherence and/or drug clearance to further guide dose escalation or de-escalations dependent on the 6-TG concentration. The reactive TDM for this class of medication was further supported by the publication of the range 6-TG concentrations that were associated with clinical response.[22]

As tracking 6-mercaptopurine metabolites became globally accepted, clinicians began to slowly adopt this practice for anti-TNF biologics. Soon, with increased use of reactive TDM to assess drug concentrations, therapeutic targets (ranges) for the anti-TNF biologics were soon established for adults with IBD.[15,25]

The first anti-TNF population PK study to include children occurred in those receiving infliximab in combination with an IMM in the REACH clinical trial.[10] Combining the REACH PK study with the adult infliximab clinical trial (ACCENT I), Fasanmade and colleagues developed a population PK model and found low albumin and presence of ADA (as a binary predictor) led to more rapid infliximab clearance while concurrent IMM use was associated with a 14% decrease in drug clearance.[10] In a more recent real-world study of children and young adults with CD receiving mostly infliximab monotherapy, Xiong and colleagues found that drug clearance was associated with albumin, body weight, ADA (as a continuous variable), the neutrophil CD64 expression, and the erythrocyte sedimentation rate (ESR).[10] These studies suggest that baseline drug clearance, and therefore, dose selection, may be best assessed with the use of blood biomarkers.

The development of more globally accepted therapeutic concentrations for anti-TNF biologics allowed investigators to retrospectively evaluate clinical outcomes when reactive TDM was used in real-world cohorts. In children, several studies showed that both undetectable concentrations (occurring in up to 24%–31% of patients) and ADA (up to 28.5% for adalimumab and up to 68% for infliximab) were common.[4,16,26] Fortunately, reactive TDM provided the clinician with support to dose optimize the therapeutic regimens for patients with a low or undetectable trough. In addition, there was now supportive data to minimize and/or reverse ADA with either dose optimization and/or the addition of an IMM.[27,28]

Pediatric-specific Benefits of Proactive Therapeutic Drug Monitoring

As the novel biologics often receive FDA approval before large PK studies can be performed in children, it is not surprising that children who receive "standard of care" (weight-based) anti-TNF dosing regimens are at an increased risk of loss of response or immunogenicity.[2,4,16] Therefore, the concept of proactive TDM lends itself to theoretical benefits to prevent the discovery of undetectable drug concentration or ADA in the asymptomatic child. Of most concern, children that have rapid drug clearance will lead low drug levels that may further perpetuate ADA formation and lead to secondary loss of response or a severe infusion reaction.

In a large observational study of 955 pediatric and adult patients on infliximab and 655 receiving adalimumab, Kennedy and colleagues reported ADA was detected in 62.8% of those receiving infliximab and 28.5% of those receiving adalimumab.[16] In a mostly pediatric CD cohort receiving infliximab monotherapy, Xiong and colleagues reported 68% developed ADA during the first year of therapy. While most of these ADA were low (<200 ng/m in 73.6%), any level of ADA using the ECLIA method has been shown to impact drug clearance and may impact response or increase the rate of an infusion reaction.[2,4]

In children, it is clear that a "one-size-fits-all" approach with standard (labeled) anti-TNF dosing often leads to suboptimal drug exposure and subsequently, low rates of endoscopic healing.[16,26] In fact, children receiving the standard (5 mg/kg) starting dose during induction has led to a significant rate (36%–60%) of infliximab concentrations below the first infliximab maintenance PK trough target (>5 µg/mL).[4,15,29] Moreover, when investigators used PK model estimates and Bayesian forecasting, they found only 22% (11/50) of pediatric patients starting infliximab with standard dosing would maintain a drug trough level greater than 3 µg/mL during maintenance further demonstrating a need for personalized infliximab dosing strategies in children.[30] While more data is needed, proposed strategies include an induction dose selection based on baseline albumin, the inflammatory burden (ESR, deep ulcers, or extent), and/or using Bayesian estimation and model-informed precision dosing.

Current Evidence to Support Proactive Therapeutic Drug Monitoring

Historically, there have been several prospective, controlled clinical trials conducted to assess whether there is an advantage to proactive TDM over reactive TDM. As a recent systematic review noted, most of the prior trials have failed to show a clinical benefit.[31] The one exception includes a study conducted in children receiving adalimumab for CD.[32]

In the prospective clinical trial of proactive TDM versus reactive TDM, Assa and colleagues randomized 78 anti-TNF naïve children with CD who had responded to adalimumab induction to two groups.[32] One group was assigned to proactive TDM with trough concentrations measured at weeks 4, 8, and then every 8 weeks until week-72 and the other group could only receive reactive TDM for loss of response.[32] For the proactive TDM group, doses and intervals of adalimumab were instructed to be adjusted to achieve a trough concentration of 5 μg/mL.[32] Sustained steroid-free clinical remission between weeks 8 to 72 was achieved in 82% assigned to proactive TDM and in 48% in the reactive TDM group ($P = .002$).[32] Importantly, by week72, adalimumab intensification was needed in 60% and 87% in the reactive and proactive TDM groups, respectively.[32]

The positive association between the use of proactive TDM and sustained steroid-free clinical remission in the Assa and colleagues trial,[32] is directly in-line with several real-world observational studies in both pediatric and adult IBD.[18,33] In one of the larger pediatric studies, Lyles and colleagues retrospectively reviewed outcomes in children receiving either infliximab or adalimumab prior to (pre-TDM) and after the use of proactive guidelines (pro-TDM). The guidelines at this single-center study were to proactively monitor and optimize drug levels (>5 μg/mL) at the first maintenance dose and prior to the development of gastrointestinal symptoms.[18] The primary outcome was the rate of sustained steroid-free clinical remission 22 to 52 weeks from starting anti-TNF (SCR22–52) with a secondary goal to evaluate the rate of developing high titer ADA.[18] The authors found SCR22 to 52 was achieved in 42% of pre-TDM and 59% of post-TDM (risk difference of 17.6%; 95% confidence interval [CI] 5.4%–29%, $P = .0004$).[18] The adjusted risk of developing high titer ADAs was also lower in the post-TDM group (hazard ratio 0.18, 95% CI 0.09–0.35, $P<.001$).[18]

Why Have Prior (Controlled) Proactive Therapeutic Drug Monitoring Studies in Adults Failed?

As noted prior, several retrospective studies have found that proactive TDM has led to higher rates of sustained clinical remission.[18,33] Yet, most notably, two clinical trials (TAXIT and TAILOREX) conducted in adult-onset CD failed to show a meaningful difference in outcomes when their disease was managed by either proactive TDM or reactive TDM.[34,35] In the TAXIT study, all subjects were dose optimized prior to the start of the trial with an infliximab target of 3 to 7 μg/mL during maintenance therapy.[34] Although there was no difference in remission between those dosed based on symptoms versus dosing based on trough concentrations, patients with CD receiving dose optimization had improved rates of remission from 65% to 88% ($P = .02$), improvement in CRP ($P = .001$), fewer occurrences of undetectable trough concentrations (relative risk 3.7, 95% CI 1.7–8; $P<.001$) and lower risk of relapse.[34] Similarly, in the TAILOREX study, one possible explanation for no difference in the rates of sustained steroid-free clinical remission is that the targeted maintenance infliximab concentration greater than 3 μg/mL is below the current PK targets (≥ 5 μg/mL) that have been associated with more favorable outcomes.[16]

In addition, it's important to note that prior proactive TDM studies primarily focused on maintenance dosing as no clinical trial to date has yet to report on the long-term outcomes when target concentrations were achieved during induction. Therefore, there is a risk that prior trials waiting until maintenance (**Table 1**) may have missed the window of opportunity to provide optimal drug exposure and improve short and long-term outcomes. Additionally, with studies such as CALM and PRECISION,[36,37] it is becoming more evident that optimizing the biologics based on pharmacodynamic (PD) biomarkers and use of population PK modeling with Bayesian estimation will be necessary to fully assess the benefits of proactive TDM.

Table 1
Prior prospective anti-TNF (interventional) clinical trials in patients with IBD

Trial	Cohort	Drug	Endoscopic Assessment	Intervention Proactive TDM	PD Targeting	Model-informed	Maintenance Target
TAXIT[34]	Adult IBD (n = 251)	IFX	No	Yes	No	No	3–7 µg/mL
TAILOREX[35]	Adult CD (n = 122)	IFX	Yes	Yes	Yes	No	>3 µg/mL
PRECISION[37]	Adult IBD (n = 80)	IFX	No	Yes	No	Yes	3 µg/mL
PRECISION IFX[60]	Adult & Pediatric IBD (n = 180)	IFX	No	Yes	No	Yes	Dose3: 17 µg/mL Dose4: 10 µg/mL
SERENE-UC[64]	Adult UC (n = 142)	ADA	Yes	Yes	No	No	>10 µg/mL
SERENE-CD[65]	Adult CD (n = 93)	ADA	No	Yes	Yes	No	>5 µg/mL
CALM[36]	Adult CD (n = 244)	ADA	Yes	No	Yes	No	N/A
PAILOT[32]	Pediatric CD (n = 78)	ADA	No	Yes	No	No	5 µg/mL

Abbreviations: ADA, adalimumab; CD, Crohn's disease; IBD, inflammatory bowel disease; IFX, infliximab; PD, pharmacodynamic; PK, pharmacokinetic; TDM, therapeutic drug monitoring; UC, ulcerative colitis.

Establishing Therapeutic Target Concentrations for Each Biologic

Several studies have associated favorable outcomes with early achievement of PK and PD targets for each novel biologic (**Table 2**).[16,36,38] In one of the first pediatric IBD studies to assess early TDM and disease outcomes, Singh and colleagues found that patients with IBD in persistent remission at week54 had an infliximab concentration at the first maintenance dose (week14) of 4.7 µg/mL compared to a level of 2.6 µg/mL for patients who did not have persistent remission (*P* = .03).[39] Moreover, in a cohort of 72 patients with CD, Clarkston and colleagues found that an infusion3 (week6) level ≥15.9 µg/mL was strongly associated with clinical response (area under the receiver curve [AUC] 0.73, 95% CI 0.6–0.86) while a week6 level ≥18 was associated with a start of maintenance (week14) concentration greater than 5 µg/mL (AUC 0.85, 95% CI 0.72–0.98).[15] In this study, predictors for a week6 level less than 18 µg/mL included a low body mass index (BMI), elevated ESR and c-reactive protein, low serum albumin and prednisone exposure during induction.[15] Similar trough concentrations are endorsed in the 2020 ECCO/ESPGHAN CD guidelines on TDM with recommendations to target a week2 concentration of greater than 29 µg/mL and week6 concentration greater than 18 µg/mL in order to achieve a week14 goal of greater than 5 µg/mL.[40]

Not only are early induction concentrations likely vital to the success of the anti-TNF biologics, achievement of early maintenance targets may also be the key to sustained durability. In a multivariate analysis of the PANTS cohort, Kennedy and colleagues found that the only independent factor that was associated with primary non-response was a low drug concentration at week14. The optimal week14 concentration associated with remission at week14 and week52 was 7 µg/mL for infliximab and 12 µg/mL for adalimumab.[16]

For patients with UC, Huang and colleagues found infliximab trough concentrations between 3 and 7 µg/mL during maintenance were associated with improved response rates,[41] with similar results subsequently published by Vande Casteele and colleagues[25] Multiple PK factors have also been identified to be associated with increased infliximab clearance in patients with acute severe UC, further supporting the critical need to incorporate clinical factors, baseline biomarkers of drug clearance and PD assessments when making key dose and interval selections for children hospitalized with acute, severe UC.[42]

As prior studies have shown superior outcomes with the use of combination anti-TNF and IMM,[28] combination therapy in adults with IBD quickly became the preferred treatment approach. Although rare, combination anti-TNF and 6-mercaptourine use in children has been associated with hepatosplenic T-cell lymphoma.[43] As such, it is encouraging that a post-host analysis of the SONIC trial found the superior rates of

Table 2		
Target drug (trough) concentrations for biologics		
Drug	**Timeframe**	**Target Drug Concentration**
Infliximab	Induction (week 6)	>15–18 µg/mL[15,40]
	Maintenance	>5–10 µg/mL[15,39,41]
Adalimumab	Maintenance	>8–12 µg/mL[16,45]
Vedolizumab	Induction (week 6)	>22–25 µg/mL[51,54]
	Post-Induction (week 14)	>14 µg/mL[50,54]
	Maintenance during remission	>12–20 µg/mL[13,52]
Ustekinumab	Maintenance	>5 µg/mL[56]

endoscopic healing with combination therapy were likely secondary to achieving higher anti-TNF concentrations.[38]

Therapeutic Trough Targets for Select Outcomes

As endoscopic healing has been associated with improved long-term outcomes,[44] Ungar and colleagues and others have shown that an infliximab trough of 6 to 10 µg/mL and an adalimumab trough of 8 to 12 µg/mL have been associated with endoscopic healing.[45] For patients with perianal CD, a higher target range of 10 to 15 µg/mL may be necessary as a median trough of 12.7 µg/mL was associated with perianal fistula healing.[46] Finally, for acute severe UC, an assessment of the current drug clearance (L/h) may be as important as drug exposure.[12] While the ARCH study that included 38 children with acute, severe UC failed to identify a specific cut point (target concentration) for infliximab to achieve either day7 clinical response or week8 clinical remission, Whaley and colleagues did find a day3 infliximab clearance greater than 0.02 L/h was associated with the need for colectomy (hazard ratio 58.2, 95% CI 6–568.6, $P<.001$).[42]

Vedolizumab Trough Targets

Vedolizumab is FDA-approved for use in adult-onset IBD and targets the $\alpha4\beta7$ integrin.[47,48] Prior clinical trials in adults helped establish population PK models for vedolizumab and have found that drug clearance is associated with serum albumin, extreme high body weight (>120 kg), antibodies to vedolizumab and prior anti-TNF exposure.[49,50] As vedolizumab trials in children are still ongoing, vedolizumab is largely used in children with moderate to severe IBD who have failed anti-TNF.

Hanzel and colleagues described in a prospective cohort of 51 adult patients with IBD that a threshold of greater than 22 µg/mL after induction at week6 was predictive of both mucosal healing and clinical remission. A cut-off of greater than 8 µg/mL at week22 was similarly predictive of these improved outcomes.[51] Finally, in a cohort that included adults and children, a maintenance threshold of greater than 11.5 µg/mL was also associated a higher likelihood of achieving CS-free remission.[52]

More recent studies have shown that a week6 (dose3) trough of greater than 25 µg/mL and a week14 (dose4) greater than 14 µg/mL were associated with improved clinical remission.[53,54] Similarly, in a cohort that included mostly children, Colman and colleagues found an infusion3 (week6) trough ≥37 µg/mL and infusion4 (week14) trough ≥20 µg/mL were associated with steroid-free clinical remission at the start of maintenance (dose4).[13] In addition, the team found an inadequate drug exposure during induction (area under the concentration curve <134,580 µg*h/mL) was associated with clinical nonresponse.[13] Pre-treatment risks for poor drug exposure during induction were higher body weight (kg), an elevated inflammatory biomarker (neutrophil CD64 expression), and lower weight-based dosing (mg/kg).[13]

Ustekinumab Trough Targets

Ustekinumab is effective in adult-onset CD[55] with more recent real-world data showing efficacy in children who were refractory to anti-TNF.[14] In one of the first studies to assess ustekinumab trough concentration and treatment outcomes, Battat and colleagues found the mean trough concentration in patients with endoscopic response at week26 was 4.7 µg/mL compared to 3.8 µg/mL ($P = .03$) in nonresponders.[56] In a population PK study in adult-onset patients with UC enrolled in a phase III trial, Xu and colleagues found body weight, baseline serum albumin, gender and antibodies to ustekinumab were covariates for ustekinumab clearance.[57] Finally, they found that the 6 mg/kg intravenous induction dose and the 90 mg subcutaneous dose every 8 weeks (maintenance) provided optimal exposure-response.[57]

Despite these promising results, no real-world pediatric-specific PK study for ustekinumab has been published to date. In Phase 1, 16-week induction dosing ranging study (UniStar), Rosh and colleagues found that the ustekinumab PK in children was similar to adults with CD but the serum ustekinumab concentrations were lower among those with a body weight less than 40 kg as compared with patients ≥40 kg.[12] Moreover, in a retrospective review of children receiving ustekinumab, Dayan and colleagues found that dose escalation (62% of the cohort) and re-induction was common.[14] Similar to other biologics used for pediatric CD, these data suggest ustekinumab PK in children may be distinct from adults and uncovered a significant knowledge gap for dose optimization for this class of biologics.

Application of Therapeutic Drug Monitoring in the Real-World: Pharmacokinetics Dashboards

Emerging data have described multiple PK factors affecting drug concentrations with biologic therapy, including weight, age, serum albumin, disease activity, ADA and inflammatory markers including CRP, ESR, and neutrophil CD64 expression.[10,30,58] Given the PK variability of the anti-TNF biologics in children and multiple biomarkers of anti-TNF clearance, novel PK dashboards (clinical decision support tools) have been developed.[4,59] The PK dashboards incorporate past drug administrations, account for biomarkers of drug clearance and use a population PK model with Bayesian estimation to forecast future drug concentrations.[4,59] In order to increase everyday use and avoid trial and error dose intensifications that may delay the time to achieve targeted drug concentrations, a PK dashboard has now been integrated within the electronic health record.[4]

The PRECISION trial was the first randomized control trial to evaluate the effectiveness of model-informed dosing (with a PK dashboard) in adults with IBD on infliximab. In this study, patients with IBD receiving maintenance infliximab were continued on a standard of care or dose optimized with a PK dashboard.[37] After 1 year, subjects receiving model-informed dosing to maintain a trough greater than 3 µg/mL had lower rates of loss of response to infliximab as well as lower median fecal calprotectin at 1 year.[37]

Similarly to the PRECISION trial's application of a PK dashboard for maintenance therapy with infliximab, Dubinsky and colleagues demonstrated that the proactive application of a PK dashboard during infliximab induction led to improved clinical outcomes and reduced immunogencity. In their pediatric and adult IBD cohort, the PK dashboard (relying on individual laboratory and dosing data) recommended accelerated dosing for a significant number of patients (41% for third infliximab infusion and 69% for fourth infliximab infusion). Additionally, use of the dashboard was associated with a low rate of immunogenicity with less than 12.7% developing anti-drug antibodies, many of these being transient. Most importantly, 67% of the cohort remaining on infliximab at infusion4 were in steroid-free clinically remission.[60]

While there have been limited clinical trials using PK dashboards to provide model-informed dosing for children, there are two ongoing studies that should provide further insight. In a study of patients greater than 16 years of age, the OPTIMIZE trial will evaluate the efficacy and safety of personalizing infliximab regimens with proactive TDM and a PK dashboard in patients with moderately to severe CD (NCT04835506).[61] In the REMODEL-CD study, researchers are investigating the safety and effectiveness of personalized dosing of infliximab with specific PK and PD targets from the start of therapy using a PK dashboard for children and young adults with CD (NCT05660746).

DISCUSSION

Whether proactive or reactive, TDM use in both children and adults has led to improved drug durability and enhanced treatment response. While only one controlled, prospective study to date supports proactive TDM, proponents of proactive TDM have previously noted the limitations of past (negative) trials.

In a recent systematic review, which included 9 trials (8 in adults and 1 in children), Nguyen and colleagues found there was no significant difference in risk of failing to maintain clinical remission for patients who received proactive TDM (combined 38%) versus conventional management (combined 42%) with a relative risk of 0.96 (95% CI 0.81–1.13).[31] They also found there were no differences in developing ADA between the two groups.[31] As previously mentioned, the clinical landscape of proactive TDM has significantly changed since most of these studies were conducted including the type of assay used, the targeted trough concentrations, the timing of TDM, the process of dose optimizations and whether endoscopic assessments were conducted during the study. Most importantly, in the only controlled trial of proactive versus reactive TDM performed in children, Assa and colleagues found superior outcomes in those randomized to proactive TDM management further emphasizing the unique PK parameters of biologics in children.[32]

While we did not directly address the novel association between HLA haplotypes and ADA first described by Sazonovs and colleagues, it is also key to defer any conclusions until further studies are complete.[62] In their post-hoc analysis of the PANTS cohort, Sazonovs and colleagues reported that the presence of HLA-DQA1*05 allele was associated with a higher risk of immunogenicity among patients treated with infliximab or adalimumab.[62] As this cohort included predominantly patients of Western European decent, more data is needed.

Interestingly, this HLA association with ADA has not been identified in pediatric studies. In a post-hoc analysis of the PRECISION infliximab trial, immunogenicity was more prevalent in patients who did not reach the targeted drug concentrations during induction with the authors concluding that the achievement of therapeutic drug concentrations may nullify any effect of the HLA-DQA1*05 haplotype.[63] Similarly, in a cohort of mostly children with a high rate (68%) of ADA, Colman and colleagues did not find an association between HLA-DQA1*05 genotype and infliximab ADA.[2]

KEY NEXT STEPS

For the foreseeable future, it's likely that all novel biologics or small molecules receiving FDA approval for adults with IBD will continue to be used "off-label" in children until more innovative clinical trials in children can be conducted in parallel. Therefore, it will be key to continue to develop data-rich, large, prospective cohort studies to gather real-world PK and PD data to assess the safety and effectiveness of these medications in children. While the current drug concentration targets are similar for both adults and children, it is clear that "standard" adult dosing regimens are not sufficient to consistently achieve these therapeutic concentrations. Lastly, TDM should not be viewed as a zero-sum game. Based on the clinical context, it's more likely that paired together, the use of both proactive and reactive TDM will lead to improved drug durability and better long-term outcomes.

As novel biologics are FDA approved, it will be key to identify novel biomarkers of drug clearance and conduct real-world studies to identify exposure targets for distinct populations, including the very young IBD patient, patients less than 30 kg, acute severe UC and those with complicated perianal CD. Moreover, as drug exposure is optimized, it will be equally important to determine the specific therapeutic range for the individual patient. For instance, patients with more mild disease may achieve endoscopic healing with an infliximab level of 5 to 10 μg/mL, while other patients with more extensive IBD or a young age may require an anti-TNF level of 7.5 to 12.5 μg/mL or 10 to 15 μg/mL to achieve endoscopic healing.

SUMMARY

IBD has a significant impact on children. Early and sustainable interventions are needed to dose optimize the novel biologics in children as multiple studies have shown that subsets of children have a very different PK profile compared to adult-onset IBD. With the current gap in FDA-approved treatments for children, future studies should be designed to better characterize the unique PK of young children receiving these novel therapies along with thoughtful design of interventional trials that embrace modern drug optimization strategies (proactive TDM and current trough targets) and clinical practices (intensification during induction). Although more data is needed, biologic optimization may only achieved with the use of a treat-to-target precision care (T2T-PC) paradigm that includes the combination of model-informed dosing with PK dashboards, proactive TDM, and the routine use of PD monitoring.

CLINICS CARE POINTS

- Both reactive and proactive therapeutic drug monitoring have improved drug durability in children.
- Children receiving biologics demonstrate significant pharmacokinetic differences than adults. These variances may be best accounted for with the use of routine, proactive TDM and other pharmacodynamic assessments.
- Real-world evidence is providing therapeutic targets for novel biologics. It is key for the clinician to consider these updated trough targets when interpreting results of therapeutic drug monitoring.

DISCLOSURE

The authors have nothing to disclose.

FUNDING

This work was supported by the National Institutes of Health, United States (R01DK132408 to P. Minar and T32DK007727 to A. Nasr).

REFERENCES

1. Dahlhamer JM, Zammitti EP, Ward BW, et al. Prevalence of Inflammatory Bowel Disease Among Adults Aged >/=18 Years - United States, 2015. MMWR Morb Mortal Wkly Rep 2016;65(42):1166–9.
2. Colman RJ, Xiong Y, Mizuno T, et al. Antibodies-to-infliximab accelerate clearance while dose intensification reverses immunogenicity and recaptures clinical response in paediatric Crohn's disease. Aliment Pharmacol Ther 2022;55(5): 593–603.
3. Cosnes J, Gower-Rousseau C, Seksik P, et al. Epidemiology and natural history of inflammatory bowel diseases. Research Support, Non-U.S. Gov't. Gastroenterology 2011;140(6):1785–94.

4. Xiong Y, Mizuno T, Colman R, et al. Real-World Infliximab Pharmacokinetic Study Informs an Electronic Health Record-Embedded Dashboard to Guide Precision Dosing in Children with Crohn's Disease. Clin Pharmacol Ther 2021;109(6): 1639–47.

5. Colombel JF, Narula N, Peyrin-Biroulet L. Management Strategies to Improve Outcomes of Patients With Inflammatory Bowel Diseases. Gastroenterology 2017; 152(2):351–361 e5.

6. Pineton de Chambrun G, Peyrin-Biroulet L, Lemann M, et al. Clinical implications of mucosal healing for the management of IBD. Nat Rev Gastroenterol Hepatol 2010;7(1):15–29.

7. Prefontaine E, Sutherland LR, Macdonald JK, et al. Azathioprine or 6-mercaptopurine for maintenance of remission in Crohn's disease. Cochrane Database Syst Rev 2009;1:CD000067.

8. Hyams J, Crandall W, Kugathasan S, et al. Induction and maintenance infliximab therapy for the treatment of moderate-to-severe Crohn's disease in children. Multicenter Study Randomized Controlled Trial. Gastroenterology 2007;132(3): 863–73 [quiz: 1165–6].

9. Hyams J, Damaraju L, Blank M, et al. Induction and maintenance therapy with infliximab for children with moderate to severe ulcerative colitis. Randomized Controlled Trial. Clin Gastroenterol Hepatol 2012;10(4):391–399 e1.

10. Fasanmade AA, Adedokun OJ, Blank M, et al. Pharmacokinetic properties of infliximab in children and adults with Crohn's disease: a retrospective analysis of data from 2 phase III clinical trials. Clin Ther 2011;33(7):946–64.

11. Hyams JS, Turner D, Cohen SA, et al. Pharmacokinetics, Safety and Efficacy of Intravenous Vedolizumab in Paediatric Patients with Ulcerative Colitis or Crohn's Disease: Results from the Phase 2 HUBBLE Study. J Crohns Colitis 2022;16(8): 1243–54.

12. Rosh JR, Turner D, Griffiths A, et al. Ustekinumab in Paediatric Patients with Moderately to Severely Active Crohn's Disease: Pharmacokinetics, Safety, and Efficacy Results from UniStar, a Phase 1 Study. J Crohns Colitis 2021;15(11): 1931–42.

13. Colman RJ, Mizuno T, Fukushima K, et al. Real world population pharmacokinetic study in children and young adults with inflammatory bowel disease discovers novel blood and stool microbial predictors of vedolizumab clearance. Aliment Pharmacol Ther 2022. https://doi.org/10.1111/apt.17277.

14. Dayan JR, Dolinger M, Benkov K, et al. Real World Experience With Ustekinumab in Children and Young Adults at a Tertiary Care Pediatric Inflammatory Bowel Disease Center. J Pediatr Gastroenterol Nutr 2019;69(1):61–7.

15. Clarkston K, Tsai YT, Jackson K, et al. Development of Infliximab Target Concentrations During Induction in Pediatric Crohn Disease Patients. J Pediatr Gastroenterol Nutr 2019;69(1):68–74.

16. Kennedy NA, Heap GA, Green HD, et al. Predictors of anti-TNF treatment failure in anti-TNF-naive patients with active luminal Crohn's disease: a prospective, multicentre, cohort study. Lancet Gastroenterol Hepatol 2019;4(5):341–53.

17. Assa A, Dorfman L, Shouval DS, et al. Therapeutic Drug Monitoring-guided High-dose Infliximab for Infantile-onset Inflammatory Bowel Disease: A Case Series. J Pediatr Gastroenterol Nutr 2020;71(4):516–20.

18. Lyles JL, Mulgund AA, Bauman LE, et al. Effect of a Practice-wide Anti-TNF Proactive Therapeutic Drug Monitoring Program on Outcomes in Pediatric Patients with Inflammatory Bowel Disease. Inflamm Bowel Dis 2021;27(4):482–92.

19. Feuerstein JD, Nguyen GC, Kupfer SS, et al. American Gastroenterological Association Institute Clinical Guidelines C. American Gastroenterological Association Institute Guideline on Therapeutic Drug Monitoring in Inflammatory Bowel Disease. Gastroenterology 2017;153(3):827–34.

20. Jelliffe RW, Schumitzky A, Bayard D, et al. Model-based, goal-oriented, individualised drug therapy. Linkage of population modelling, new 'multiple model' dosage design, bayesian feedback and individualised target goals. Clin Pharmacokinet 1998;34(1):57–77.

21. Størset E, Åsberg A, Skauby M, et al. Improved Tacrolimus Target Concentration Achievement Using Computerized Dosing in Renal Transplant Recipients–A Prospective, Randomized Study. Transplantation 2015;99(10):2158–66.

22. Dubinsky MC, Lamothe S, Yang HY, et al. Pharmacogenomics and metabolite measurement for 6-mercaptopurine therapy in inflammatory bowel disease. Gastroenterology 2000;118(4):705–13.

23. Papamichael K, Clarke WT, Vande Casteele N, et al. Comparison of Assays for Therapeutic Monitoring of Infliximab and Adalimumab in Patients With Inflammatory Bowel Diseases. Clin Gastroenterol Hepatol 2021;19(4):839–41.e2.

24. Steenholdt C, Ainsworth MA, Tovey M, et al. Comparison of Techniques for Monitoring Infliximab and Antibodies Against Infliximab in Crohn's Disease. Ther Drug Monit 2013;35(4):530–8.

25. Vande Casteele N, Ferrante M, Van Assche G, et al. Trough concentrations of infliximab guide dosing for patients with inflammatory bowel disease. Gastroenterology 2015;148(7):1320–9.e3.

26. Minar P, Saeed SA, Afreen M, et al. Practical Use of Infliximab Concentration Monitoring in Pediatric Crohn Disease. J Pediatr Gastroenterol Nutr 2016;62(5):715–22.

27. Colman RJ, Portocarrero-Castillo A, Chona D, et al. Favorable Outcomes and Anti-TNF Durability After Addition of an Immunomodulator for Anti-Drug Antibodies in Pediatric IBD Patients. Inflamm Bowel Dis 2021;27(4):507–15.

28. Colombel JF, Sandborn WJ, Reinisch W, et al. Infliximab, azathioprine, or combination therapy for Crohn's disease. Comparative Study Multicenter Study Randomized Controlled Trial Research Support, Non-U.S. Gov't. N Engl J Med 2010;362(15):1383–95.

29. Guido AJ, Crandall W, Homan E, et al. Improving Post-induction Antitumor Necrosis Factor Therapeutic Drug Monitoring in Pediatric Inflammatory Bowel Disease. J Pediatr Gastroenterol Nutr 2020;70(1):48–54.

30. Dubinsky MC, Phan BL, Singh N, et al. Pharmacokinetic Dashboard-Recommended Dosing Is Different than Standard of Care Dosing in Infliximab-Treated Pediatric IBD Patients. AAPS J 2017;19(1):215–22.

31. Nguyen NH, Solitano V, Vuyyuru SK, et al. Proactive Therapeutic Drug Monitoring Versus Conventional Management for Inflammatory Bowel Diseases: A Systematic Review and Meta-Analysis. Gastroenterology 2022;163(4):937–49.e2.

32. Assa A, Matar M, Turner D, et al. Proactive Monitoring of Adalimumab Trough Concentration Associated With Increased Clinical Remission in Children With Crohn's Disease Compared With Reactive Monitoring. Gastroenterology 2019;157(4):985–996 e2.

33. Papamichael K, Chachu KA, Vajravelu RK, et al. Improved Long-term Outcomes of Patients With Inflammatory Bowel Disease Receiving Proactive Compared With Reactive Monitoring of Serum Concentrations of Infliximab. Clin Gastroenterol Hepatol 2017;15(10):1580–1588 e3.

34. Vande Casteele N, Compernolle G, Ballet V, et al. Results on the Optimisation Phase of the Prospective Controlled Trough Level Adapted Infliximab Treatment (TAXIT) Trial. Gastroenterology 2012;142(5):S211–2.

35. D'Haens G, Vermeire S, Lambrecht G, et al. Increasing Infliximab Dose Based on Symptoms, Biomarkers, and Serum Drug Concentrations Does Not Increase Clinical, Endoscopic, and Corticosteroid-Free Remission in Patients With Active Luminal Crohn's Disease. Gastroenterology 2018;154(5):1343–51. e1.

36. Colombel JF, Panaccione R, Bossuyt P, et al. Effect of tight control management on Crohn's disease (CALM): a multicentre, randomised, controlled phase 3 trial. Lancet 2018;390(10114):2779–89.

37. Strik AS, Lowenberg M, Mould DR, et al. Efficacy of dashboard driven dosing of infliximab in inflammatory bowel disease patients; a randomized controlled trial. Scand J Gastroenterol 2021;56(2):145–54.

38. Colombel JF, Adedokun OJ, Gasink C, et al. Combination Therapy With Infliximab and Azathioprine Improves Infliximab Pharmacokinetic Features and Efficacy: A Post Hoc Analysis. Clin Gastroenterol Hepatol 2019;17(8):1525–32.e1.

39. Singh N, Rosenthal CJ, Melmed GY, et al. Early infliximab trough levels are associated with persistent remission in pediatric patients with inflammatory bowel disease. Inflamm Bowel Dis 2014;20(10):1708–13.

40. van Rheenen PF, Aloi M, Assa A, et al. The Medical Management of Paediatric Crohn's Disease: an ECCO-ESPGHAN Guideline Update. J Crohns Colitis 2020. https://doi.org/10.1093/ecco-jcc/jjaa161.

41. Huang VW, Prosser C, Kroeker KI, et al. Knowledge of Fecal Calprotectin and Infliximab Trough Levels Alters Clinical Decision-making for IBD Outpatients on Maintenance Infliximab Therapy. Inflamm Bowel Dis 2015;21(6):1359–67.

42. Whaley KG, Xiong Y, Karns R, et al. Multicenter Cohort Study of Infliximab Pharmacokinetics and Therapy Response in Pediatric Acute Severe Ulcerative Colitis. Clin Gastroenterol Hepatol 2022. https://doi.org/10.1016/j.cgh.2022.08.016.

43. Shah ED, Coburn ES, Nayyar A, et al. Systematic review: hepatosplenic T-cell lymphoma on biologic therapy for inflammatory bowel disease, including data from the Food and Drug Administration Adverse Event Reporting System. Aliment Pharmacol Ther 2020;51(5):527–33.

44. Ungaro RC, Yzet C, Bossuyt P, et al. Deep Remission at 1 Year Prevents Progression of Early Crohn's Disease. Gastroenterology 2020;159(1):139–47.

45. Ungar B, Levy I, Yavne Y, et al. Optimizing Anti-TNF-alpha Therapy: Serum Levels of Infliximab and Adalimumab Are Associated With Mucosal Healing in Patients With Inflammatory Bowel Diseases. Clin Gastroenterol Hepatol 2016;14(4):550–557 e2.

46. El-Matary W, Walters TD, Huynh HQ, et al. Higher Postinduction Infliximab Serum Trough Levels Are Associated With Healing of Fistulizing Perianal Crohn's Disease in Children. Inflamm Bowel Dis 2019;25(1):150–5.

47. Feagan BG, Rutgeerts P, Sands BE, et al. Vedolizumab as Induction and Maintenance Therapy for Ulcerative Colitis. N Engl J Med 2013;369(8):699–710.

48. Sandborn WJ, Feagan BG, Rutgeerts P, et al. Vedolizumab as Induction and Maintenance Therapy for Crohn's Disease. N Engl J Med 2013;369(8):711–21.

49. Hanzel J, Dreesen E, Vermeire S, et al. Pharmacokinetic-Pharmacodynamic Model of Vedolizumab for Targeting Endoscopic Remission in Patients With Crohn Disease: Posthoc Analysis of the LOVE-CD Study. Inflamm Bowel Dis 2021. https://doi.org/10.1093/ibd/izab143.

50. Rosario M, Dirks NL, Gastonguay MR, et al. Population pharmacokinetics-pharmacodynamics of vedolizumab in patients with ulcerative colitis and Crohn's disease. Aliment Pharmacol Ther 2015;42(2):188–202.

51. Hanzel J, Sever N, Ferkolj I, et al. Early vedolizumab trough levels predict combined endoscopic and clinical remission in inflammatory bowel disease. United European Gastroenterol J 2019;7(6):741–9.
52. Ungaro RC, Yarur A, Jossen J, et al. Higher Trough Vedolizumab Concentrations During Maintenance Therapy are Associated With Corticosteroid-Free Remission in Inflammatory Bowel Disease. J Crohns Colitis 2019;13(8):963–9.
53. Singh S, Dulai PS, Vande Casteele N, et al. Systematic review with meta-analysis: association between vedolizumab trough concentration and clinical outcomes in patients with inflammatory bowel diseases. Aliment Pharmacol Ther 2019;50(8): 848–57.
54. Restellini S, Afif W. Update on TDM (Therapeutic Drug Monitoring) with Ustekinumab, Vedolizumab and Tofacitinib in Inflammatory Bowel Disease. J Clin Med 2021;10(6). https://doi.org/10.3390/jcm10061242.
55. Feagan BG, Sandborn WJ, Gasink C, et al. Ustekinumab as Induction and Maintenance Therapy for Crohn's Disease. N Engl J Med 2016;375(20):1946–60.
56. Battat R, Kopylov U, Bessissow T, et al. Association Between Ustekinumab Trough Concentrations and Clinical, Biomarker, and Endoscopic Outcomes in Patients With Crohn's Disease. Clin Gastroenterol Hepatol 2017;15(9):1427–34.e2.
57. Xu Y, Hu C, Chen Y, et al. Population Pharmacokinetics and Exposure-Response Modeling Analyses of Ustekinumab in Adults With Moderately to Severely Active Ulcerative Colitis. J Clin Pharmacol 2020;60(7):889–902.
58. Winter DA, Joosse ME, de Wildt SN, et al. Pharmacokinetics, Pharmacodynamics, and Immunogenicity of Infliximab in Pediatric Inflammatory Bowel Disease: A Systematic Review and Revised Dosing Considerations. J Pediatr Gastroenterol Nutr 2020;70(6):763–76.
59. Mould DR, D'Haens G, Upton RN. Clinical Decision Support Tools: The Evolution of a Revolution. Clin Pharmacol Ther 2016;99(4):405–18.
60. Dubinsky MC, Mendiolaza ML, Phan BL, et al. Dashboard-Driven Accelerated Infliximab Induction Dosing Increases Infliximab Durability and Reduces Immunogenicity. Inflamm Bowel Dis 2022;28(9):1375–85.
61. Papamichael K, Jairath V, Zou G, et al. Proactive infliximab optimisation using a pharmacokinetic dashboard versus standard of care in patients with Crohn's disease: study protocol for a randomised, controlled, multicentre, open-label study (the OPTIMIZE trial). BMJ Open 2022;12(4):e057656.
62. Sazonovs A, Kennedy NA, Moutsianas L, et al. HLA-DQA1*05 Carriage Associated With Development of Anti-Drug Antibodies to Infliximab and Adalimumab in Patients With Crohn's Disease. Gastroenterology 2020;158(1):189–99.
63. Spencer EA, Stachelski J, Dervieux T, et al. Failure to Achieve Target Drug Concentrations During Induction and Not HLA-DQA1 *05 Carriage Is Associated With Antidrug Antibody Formation in Patients With Inflammatory Bowel Disease. Gastroenterology 2022;162(6):1746–1748 e3.
64. Colombel J-F, Panés J, D'Haens GR, et al. Therapeutic Drug Monitoring Dosing Regimen With Adalimumab in Patients with Moderately to Severe Active Ulcerative Colitis: Results from the SERENE-UC Maintenance Study. Am J Gastroenterol 2020;S454.
65. D'Haens GR, Sandborn WJ, Loftus EV, et al. Higher vs Standard Adalimumab Induction Dosing Regimens and Two Maintenance Strategies: Randomized SERENE CD Trial Results. Gastroenterology 2022;162(7):1876–90.

The Role of Diet in Pediatric Inflammatory Bowel Disease

Lindsey Albenberg, DO

KEYWORDS

- Inflammatory bowel disease • Exclusive enteral nutrition
- Crohn's disease exclusion diet • Microbiome

KEY POINTS

- Diet is an environmental risk factor that has been linked to inflammatory bowel disease (IBD) pathogenesis and is important to consider as a therapeutic target because it is modifiable.
- Exclusive enteral nutrition has been used in the treatment of children with Crohn's disease for many years, and multiple studies have demonstrated efficacy, particularly for the induction of remission.
- The Crohn's disease exclusion diet can be used as an alternative to exclusive enteral nutrition for the induction of remission and may be more acceptable to patients.
- Diet is important to IBD patients and can be used to reduce inflammation, improve symptoms, and/or enhance general health and physicians should provide evidence-based guidance.

INTRODUCTION

The pathogenesis of inflammatory bowel disease (IBD) is complex with both genetic and environmental contributions. Advances in DNA sequencing technology have allowed the identification of 240 genetic polymorphisms that are associated with the risk for the development of IBD.[1] However, in total, these genetic loci account for only a modest proportion of disease variance.[2] Therefore, it seems that environmental factors represent the most significant contributors to IBD pathogenesis. Among the environmental factors associated with IBD, diet and the intestinal microbiota would seem the most likely to be modifiable, making them potential targets for disease treatment. Although the relationship between diet and the gut microbiota is complex, it is clear that dietary nutrients can directly regulate immune function and can modify the composition of the gut microbiota and their production of biologically important metabolites.

Division of Gastroenterology, Hepatology, and Nutrition, Children's Hospital of Philadelphia, Perelman School of Medicine at the University of Pennsylvania, 2716 South Street, 14-140, Philadelphia, PA 19146, USA
E-mail address: albenbergl@chop.edu

Gastroenterol Clin N Am 52 (2023) 565–577
https://doi.org/10.1016/j.gtc.2023.05.011
0889-8553/23/© 2023 Elsevier Inc. All rights reserved.

Thus far, our therapeutic approach in IBD has focused on targeted biologic and small molecule therapies. However, increasingly, attention is being placed on diet not only for its ability to correct nutritional deficiencies and support adequate weight gain and linear growth but also as a potential therapy based on what we know of the epidemiology of IBD and diet's ability to alter innate immunity and affect mucosal barrier function. In addition, despite significant advances in the development of pharmacologic therapies for the treatment of IBD as well as an improved understanding of their pharmacokinetics, the current approaches to treatment remain suboptimal.[3] It is clear that there is a need to explore therapies with alternative mechanisms, such as diet, as either primary or adjunctive treatment. This approach has many important, potential advantages including reducing exposure to medications while targeting the environmental mechanism of disease without additional toxicity which could be especially important for children and adolescents where disease is expected to be long lasting.

DIET AND DEVELOPMENT OF INFLAMMATORY BOWEL DISEASE

Since the twentieth century, there has been a dramatic global increase in the incidence and prevalence of IBD. The highest incidence and prevalence are in North America and Europe, and the incidence is increasing in parts of the world where IBD was once rare.[4] The reasons for this are likely multifactorial, but again parallel industrialization with newly industrialized countries reporting rapid increases in the incidence of IBD.[5] This trend is too fast to be explained by genetics alone suggesting a link between lifestyle "Westernization" and an increase in IBD incidence. Diet is one of the more obvious environmental changes linked with industrialization. Indeed, with industrialization came the introduction of foods not previously commonly consumed such as dairy, refined sugars, refined vegetable oils, and cereals, among others.[6]

Numerous observational studies have demonstrated an association between Western dietary patterns and an increase in IBD risk. In a systematic review to evaluate the association between prediagnosis intake of nutrients and food groups and the risk of subsequent IBD diagnosis, high dietary intakes of total fats, polyunsaturated fatty acids, omega-6 fatty acids, and meat were associated with an increased risk of Crohn's disease (CD) and ulcerative colitis (UC).[7] High fiber and fruit intakes were associated with decreased CD risk, and high vegetable intake was associated with decreased UC risk. Similarly, the association between fiber intake and incident IBD was examined in the large, prospective Nurses' Health Study. Healthy nurses consuming large amounts of fiber were 40% less likely to be subsequently diagnosed with CD, and no association was observed for UC.[8] More recently, food frequency questionnaires from three large prospective cohort studies, including the Nurses' Health Study, were assessed to evaluate the overall inflammatory potential of the diet and risk of IBD.[9] Lo and colleagues used the empirical dietary inflammatory pattern (EDIP) score which is a weighted sum of 18 food groups with higher EDIP scores, previously associated with higher serum inflammatory markers, corresponding to a more pro-inflammatory diet. They found that healthy adults with EDIP scores in the highest quartile had a 51% increased risk of developing CD. In this study, they also did not identify an association between EDIP score and development of UC potentially suggesting differences in environmental risk factors or the contributions of these risk factors in these diseases. Importantly, higher intake of ultra-processed food was recently associated with risk of *both* CD and UC in a prospective cohort study of more than 100,000 participants from 21 countries.[10] Further studies are needed to determine the contribution of specific foods or nutrients, the processing of specific foods, and overall dietary pattern to the pathogenesis of IBD.

PATIENT AND PARENT CONCERN ABOUT DIET

It is well recognized that diet is very important to our patients. "What should my child eat?" is one of the first questions that parents of children diagnosed with IBD ask their providers. It has been shown across several studies conducted in multiple countries that approximately 60% of adult patients with IBD modify their diet, avoiding foods that they believe exacerbate symptoms such as milk, spicy food, fatty food, sugary food, fruits, vegetables, alcohol, carbonated beverages, and coffee/tea.[11–13] Up to two-thirds of adult patients report depriving themselves of their favorite foods because they believe that avoiding these foods could prevent relapse.[11] Similar practices have also been observed in children. Bramuzzo and colleagues[14] administered questionnaires regarding dietary beliefs to patients with IBD ages 8 to 17 years and their parents. About 60% of patients reported dietary changes after the IBD diagnosis despite the majority reporting not following a prescribed therapeutic diet. In addition, nearly half of patients and parents believed that some foods could induce or worsen symptoms during an IBD flare and the foods reported were nearly identical to those described in adult studies. Importantly, we do not have evidence for a direct link between these restrictions and reduction in inflammation. However, expert opinion on dietary recommendations based on data in animal models and human studies for a number of these specific dietary components has been described in the International Organization for the Study of IBD (IOIBD) Guidelines,[15] but is beyond the scope of this review.

DIET AS A PRIMARY THERAPY IN PEDIATRIC PATIENTS WITH INFLAMMATORY BOWEL DISEASE
Exclusive Enteral Nutrition

Diet can be used as primary therapy for certain patients with CD. Exclusive enteral nutrition (EEN) with elemental, semi-elemental, or polymeric formula has been widely studied for the induction of remission. The efficacy of EEN for the induction of remission has been well established and has led to the recommendation that EEN be considered first line for the induction of remission in children with active, luminal CD in pediatric society IBD treatment guidelines including the European Crohn's and Colitis Organization and European Society for Pediatric Gastroenterology, Hepatology, and Nutrition (ECCO-ESPGHAN) and Porto IBD groups.[16,17] A meta-analysis which included eight trials comparing EEN and corticosteroids (CS) for the induction of remission in newly diagnosed *or* relapsed pediatric CD did not find a clinical treatment benefit of CS in either scenario.[18] In addition to symptomatic improvement, EEN has been associated with mucosal healing, which may be a superior predictor of long-term outcomes.[19,20] In a prospective, open-label trial where children with CD were randomized to receive oral CS or EEN with a polymeric formula for 10 weeks, EEN was significantly more effective than CS in healing the mucosa, as determined by both endoscopic and histologic criteria.[21] Similarly, in a recent French randomized trial that included 19 children with newly diagnosed CD, mucosal healing by Crohn's Disease Endoscopic Index of Severity was identified in 89% of the EEN group and only 17% of the CS group.[22]

The most common EEN protocol for the induction of remission involves the administration of a nutritionally complete formula at 100% of estimated caloric needs for 4 to 12 weeks to induce remission.[23] It is widely recognized that there is no major difference in efficacy of EEN based on the composition of the formula.[24] Specifically, there is no difference in remission rates when comparing non-elemental and elemental formulas, formulas of varying fat content, or formulas with different fat composition (medium or long-chain triglyceride content).[24] Formula can be consumed orally or can be administered through a nasogastric (NG) or gastrostomy tube. A retrospective review of EEN administered orally or via an overnight continuous NG infusion showed similar rates of induction of clinical remission.[25] Thus, it is recommended to initially offer EEN with a palatable formula by mouth and only introduce an NG tube if the patient is unable to drink the required amount of formula.[17]

When considering EEN, patient selection is important. EEN is not recommended for UC. The reason for this is primarily secondary to early studies demonstrating less satisfactory outcomes in patients with UC[26] or CD primarily involving the colon.[27] Further studies of EEN efficacy based on CD disease location have demonstrated variable results. Afzal and colleagues[27] performed a prospective study of EEN to induce remission in children with CD and examined rates of remission based on disease location–ileal ($n = 12$), ileocolonic ($n = 39$), or colonic ($n = 14$). Remission, defined by both clinical and endoscopic scores, was the lowest in the colonic disease only group. However, a subsequent observational study ($n = 110$) found that patients with colonic disease were *not* less likely to achieve clinical remission.[28] Thus, guidelines suggest that children with active CD that is purely inflammatory in behavior (non-penetrating, non-stricturing) regardless of disease location are eligible for EEN for the induction of remission.[17] However, in a large, multicenter, retrospective study, colonic involvement was associated with reduced adherence.[29] In this same study, age greater than 15 years and pediatric Crohn's disease activity index (PCDAI) greater than 50 were associated with lower rates of clinical remission—another consideration in patient selection.[29] Although EEN is not recommended for the treatment of UC, a recent randomized trial of standard of care (SOC) versus 7 days of EEN in addition to SOC in adults hospitalized with acute severe UC, found that patients in the EEN group had lower rates of need for salvage therapy or colectomy, shorter hospital stays, and improvements in biochemical markers of inflammation.[30] Further studies are need to explore the potential benefits of short-term adjunctive EEN in UC.

Although "exclusive" (100% of caloric needs from formula) regimens are the most widely accepted for induction of remission, there are data to support more flexible protocols with 75% to 90% of caloric needs provided from formula and the remainder provided from table foods.[31,32] Protocols which include a small amount of table food may improve EEN compliance and acceptance; however, this has not been formally studied. Although the optimal percentage of calories for the induction of remission (balancing efficacy and acceptability) has not been determined, there are data demonstrating a lack of efficacy to induce remission with partial enteral nutrition (PEN) protocols that provide 50% of calories from formula.[33,34] In a comparative effectiveness study (PLEASE study) of EEN, PEN, and anti-TNF-alpha therapy for the induction of remission in pediatric CD, PEN (mean 47% calories from table foods) improved clinical symptoms, but EEN and anti-TNF-therapy were superior for reducing mucosal inflammation as estimated by fecal calprotectin.[34]

If the percentage of calories from formula must be close to 100% for the induction of remission, perhaps PEN with 50% or greater calories, but less than 100% of calories, can maintain or prolong remission. Although the literature is scarce, there may be a role for PEN in maintaining remission. Most of this work comes from studies of partial formula consumption in combination with medications. A meta-analysis of four studies found that biologic therapy coupled with PEN was more likely to lead to sustained remission at 1 year compared with biological therapy alone.[35] However, limitations included small number of studies, most of which were retrospective, and all were from adults in the same country. Future studies are needed to determine the efficacy of PEN as a maintenance strategy for children, the percentage of calories from formula required in this setting, whether the types of table foods ingested in addition to the formula need to be regulated in any way, and the role of concomitant medications.

Although EEN has been shown to be efficacious in the treatment of CD, the mechanism of action has not been well characterized. Some hypotheses involve dietary monotony, reduction in luminal antigens and exclusion of potentially pro-inflammatory foods in the standard, Western diet, a direct beneficial effect of the formula, and changes in the gut microbiota and/or metabolome.[22,36,37] The finding that formula composition does not impact outcome opposes the hypothesis that EEN formula is delivering a substance that is beneficial to reduce inflammation. The PLEASE study demonstrated superior improvements in fecal calprotectin in the EEN group compared with the PEN group despite similar intakes of formula in both groups.[34] Patients consuming more table foods had poorer outcomes, supporting the hypothesis that the mechanism of action could involve exclusion of potentially pro-inflammatory components in the usual diet. Modulation of the gut microbiota composition or function is another proposed mechanism of action of EEN.[38-40] IBD is associated with dysbiosis or an altered composition of the gut microbiota which includes decreased bacterial diversity and increases in Proteobacteria with a reduction in Firmicutes compared with healthy controls.[41] Multiple studies have demonstrated changes in the gut microbiota with EEN treatment and the results are varied based on study design and methodology, but interestingly the most frequently reported outcome is a further decrease in bacterial diversity.[42] The changes in the gut bacterial community associated with EEN can be seen rapidly, within just 7 days of initiating therapy.[43] In addition, several studies have shown more marked effects on gut microbiota composition in patients who respond to EEN compared with those who do not respond[43,44] and it may also be possible to predict better response to EEN based on baseline microbiota composition.[40] Further work is needed to enhance our understanding of EEN mechanisms which may lead to improvements in dietary therapies or our ability to personalize therapeutic recommendations.

Pediatric patients with IBD are unique and there are specific concerns which must be addressed, including growth and skeletal health, long disease duration and subsequent desire to reduce medication exposure, and unique effects on quality of life. Overall, EEN has the ability to spare the use of CS and other immunosuppressive therapies and has the additional benefits of improvements in linear growth and bone health.[45-48] In addition, despite the psychosocial nuances of EEN, studies have generally shown improvements in quality of life in both children and adults with short-term, induction of remission protocols.[34,49,50] Quality of life has not been studied in PEN for maintenance of remission. Overall, EEN has many potential benefits, but optimal positioning needs to be considered in the biologic era where there is a reduced need for CS, as EEN has historically been positioned as an alternative to CS in induction of remission protocols. Potential opportunities include EEN in combination with pharmacologic therapies to induce remission especially with biologic medications with longer time to effect, as a bridge in the setting of delayed medication insurance approval or in patients where immunosuppression should be delayed (immunization catch up or intra-abdominal sepsis) or as a bridge to PEN or whole food-based therapeutic diets.

Crohn's Disease Exclusion Diet

Despite the effectiveness of EEN, there are clear limitations affecting acceptability and adherence including taste fatigue as well as the social implications. In a survey of CD patients treated with EEN and their families, respondents viewed EEN positively but would preferentially choose a hypothetical whole food-based alternative if offered.[51] The Crohn's disease exclusion diet (CDED) was proposed in 2014 as a potentially better tolerated alternative to EEN, combining PEN with a whole food, anti-inflammatory diet.[52] The design of the whole food portion of the diet was based on reducing exposure to foods or food additives shown to induce inflammation, alter gut barrier function, or change the microbiome in animal models or in vitro.[53] The whole food portion of the CDED is composed of mandatory, allowed, and disallowed foods. Mandatory foods include chicken breast, eggs, potatoes, apples, and bananas and their purpose is to ensure adequate sources of lean protein as well as specific fibers as substrates for production of short-chain fatty acids by the microbiota. The disallowed foods and additives include dairy, wheat, high-fat meats including red meat, and emulsifiers. The most commonly studied protocol involves two phases for induction.[53] In phase 1 (weeks 0–6), 50% of estimated calorie needs come from an oral, polymeric formula and 50% of calorie needs come from the structured, whole food-based diet. In phase 2 (weeks 6–12), formula is reduced to 25% calorie needs and the whole food portion of the diet is expanded to 75% calorie needs with foods such as starchy vegetables, legumes, and whole grains in limited amounts added. A maintenance phase has been described[54] but has not yet been extensively studied.

The first CDED report was a retrospective description of 33 children and 14 adults with active CD (either newly diagnosed or relapsed) who followed the 12-week induction of remission protocol.[52] The primary outcome, clinical remission (PCDAI <7 in children or Harvey–Bradshaw Index ≤3 in adults) at week 6, was met in 70% of children and 69% of adults and most of the cohort (84%) remained in remission at week 12. In children, baseline disease severity was a predictor of response at week 6.

In 2019, a randomized trial was published comparing the CDED + PEN protocol above to EEN for the induction of remission in 74 children with mild to moderate CD.[53] Those randomized to the EEN arm received 100% of calories from formula in phase 1 and 25% of calories from formula in phase 2 with the remainder of calories coming from a free diet. The primary outcome was tolerability which was greater in the CDED group compared with the EEN group. At week 6, there was no difference in compliance or in rate of remission. However, at week 12, once the EEN group had transitioned to 75% calories from free diet, there was a significantly higher rate of corticosteroid-free remission in the CDED group. Although fecal calprotectin reduction was seen in both groups at week 6, there seemed to be a rebound effect at week 12 in the EEN group with return to 75% free diet. It is important to note that this cohort had relatively mild disease activity with median PCDAI of 25 and 27.5 in the CDED and EEN groups, respectively. Interestingly, in a post hoc analysis of the clinical trial data, most of the clinical effect in both arms could be seen by week 3,[55] suggesting a diet-responsive phenotype which can be identified early in the course of therapy.

The efficacy of CDED for the induction of remission has also been demonstrated in adults with CD[54,56,57] including a study of CDED + PEN ($n = 20$) compared with CDED alone ($n = 24$), without formula.[54] Yanai and colleagues demonstrated that CDED with or without PEN was effective for induction (weeks 6 and 12) and maintenance (week 24) of remission in mild to moderate, uncomplicated, biologic naïve CD. Importantly, this was the only randomized trial of a dietary monotherapy to include an endoscopic outcome. All patients who had not withdrawn or received additional medication due to poor response ($n = 28$) had a colonoscopy at week 24 demonstrating endoscopic remission in 35%. Overall, the results of this trial suggest that CDED without formula can be considered in patients who do not tolerate formula. In pediatrics, dietician involvement will be critical to identify patients in whom this approach may or may not be appropriate based on anthropometrics, caloric intake, and nutritional completeness of the diet (eg, in picky eaters). CDED plus PEN will likely be the best approach for most pediatric patients. Importantly, there are also pediatric patients who may require even more formula than recommended in the traditional protocol for the same reasons described above.

Another potential role for CDED is as an adjunct to medication. Sigall-Boneh and colleagues[58] published a retrospective study of children and adults who had lost response to biologic therapy where the addition of CDED was the only change in treatment. Twenty-one patients (11 adults and 10 children) met study criteria and clinical remission by physician's global assessment and Harvey–Bradshaw Index after 6 weeks was achieved in 61.9%. Most (10/13) of the patients achieving clinical remission at week 6 continued successfully with their biologic therapy through follow-up demonstrating the potential for patients to regain remission with CDED when failing medical therapy with biologics. A case series by Scarallo and colleagues[59] also demonstrated the examples of CDED plus co-medication in children with severe CD. Prospective studies are needed, but dietary therapy could serve as an adjunct to pharmacologic therapies to induce remission in patients whose disease is partially responding or is refractory to conventional therapies.

Similar to EEN, clinical response to CDED has been associated with changes in the microbiome and the metabolome. In the pediatric randomized trial,[53] there were significant decreases in Haemophilus, Veillonella, Prevotella, and Anaerostipes with increases in Oscillibacter and Roseburia by 16S gene sequencing when comparing baseline to weeks 6 and 12 in the CDED group. Most of these same changes were observed in the EEN group with a few additional taxa increasing or decreasing with treatment. Importantly, in the EEN group, there was a rebound in these changes from week 6 to 12 with increased table food consumption, whereas changes continued in the CDED group. In addition, non-responders at week 6 exhibited less change in microbiome composition with a smaller reduction in Proteobacteria. A subsequent analysis of shotgun metagenomic sequencing data from the randomized trial participants compared with healthy controls[60] demonstrated compositional and functional changes between baseline and week 12 toward the healthy samples in both diets and suggested partial, but not complete, correction of dysbiosis. There is recent evidence that metabolic pathways may be involved in dietary therapy-induced remission such as tryptophan metabolism pathways.[61,62]

DIETS NOT CURRENTLY RECOMMENDED FOR REDUCTION OF INFLAMMATION

Other whole food-based diets have been proposed for the treatment of IBD, but none have been as well studied as CDED or have been associated with mucosal healing in high-quality studies. CD-TREAT[63] was developed to replicate EEN using whole foods by excluding gluten and lactose and matching one of the most commonly used EEN formulas in macronutrients, vitamins, minerals, and fiber. The diet is individualized based on energy requirements and food preferences. In a crossover study where 25 healthy adults were randomized to CD-TREAT or EEN for 7 days with a washout in between, CD-TREAT was easier to follow and more satiating than EEN and CD-TREAT and EEN induced similar changes on the microbiome and metabolome.[63] Subsequently, in an open label trial of five children with mild to moderate relapsed CD, 4 weeks of CD-TREAT led to improvement in PCDAI and reduction of fecal calprotectin.[63] Although efficacy needs to be replicated in a large study, CD-TREAT could be another promising alternative to EEN in the future.

The specific carbohydrate diet (SCD) involves strict exclusion of grains, most refined sugars, and processed foods and was popular with patients based on Elaine

Gottschall's book *Breaking the Viscous Cycle*[64] before acquiring scientific interest. The diet was based on the hypothesis that in the setting of intestinal inflammation, undigested disaccharides and polysaccharides travel to the colon where they promote the growth of pro-inflammatory bacteria leading to subsequent alterations in mucosal barrier function. Initially, retrospective studies and small prospective series were published, primarily in children with CD, demonstrating variable results but overall improvements in clinical and laboratory parameters.[65–68] However, larger, controlled trials were lacking. The PRODUCE study,[69] which used N-of-1 methodology to compare SCD with a modified SCD (MSCD, allowing rice and oats) to usual diet in children with IBD, demonstrated that changes in symptoms and fecal calprotectin with SCD and MSCD compared with usual diet were highly variable by individual. In addition, a high rate of withdrawal from the trial limited conclusions regarding efficacy.

In the DINE-CD trial,[70] adults with mild to moderate CD symptoms were randomized to SCD or Mediterranean diet (MD) for 12 weeks. For the first 6 weeks, participants received prepared meals and snacks and continued their assigned diet independently from weeks 6 to 12. The primary and secondary outcomes, symptomatic remission, fecal calprotectin response, and C-reactive protein (CRP) response were assessed at weeks 6 and 12. At week 6, 46.5% in the SCD group and 43.5% in the MD group achieved symptomatic remission. Rates of symptomatic remission were similar at week 12 and fecal calprotectin and CRP response were uncommon at both time points. Interestingly, the SCD was not superior to the MD for any of the primary or secondary outcomes. Overall, few patients achieved combined symptomatic remission and reduction of inflammation. Given that MD may be easier to follow than SCD and the well-described benefits of MD for general health, MD seems promising as an adjunctive therapy for patients with CD.

Although EEN and CDED have proven to be effective in inducing remission in CD, the role of diet as a potential therapy for UC remains unclear. There are no prospective, randomized trials of dietary interventions in children with UC. Based on epidemiologic data[7] and one cross-sectional study[71] demonstrating higher odds of relapse with higher red meat (particularly processed meats and sulfur) consumption in adults with UC, the IOIBD guidelines[15] recommended that patients with UC should reduce consumption of these foods. Recommendations also included reducing consumption of certain long-chain fats and additives. A small pilot study[72] of a diet low in sulfated amino acids, saturated and polyunsaturated fat, and food additives demonstrated feasibility and clinical response in children with UC, but larger studies are needed to confirm these findings.

SUMMARY

Nutrition is an important consideration in the care of children with IBD to achieve optimal health, correct nutritional deficiencies, achieve weight restoration and maintenance, and complete normative linear growth. Food and nutrition are important to patients and the available data support the hypothesis that diet can contribute to IBD risk and can play a role in regulating mucosal immune function through many mechanisms including those influenced by the gut microbiota. Many patients with IBD desire alternatives to long-term immunosuppressive therapy and there are evidence-based options for patients with additional promising options in the pipeline. EEN remains the gold standard for the induction of remission in pediatric CD, but there are challenges in acceptability. The challenges of EEN may be overcome with less limiting diets such as CDED, which has become a valuable option for children with CD. Recognizing the challenges of dietary clinical trials, adhering to high methodological standards in future studies is important. Going forward, it is also critical to better understand the mechanism of action of dietary therapies, which will inform the development of novel approaches. In clinical practice, assessing the goals of the patient and family is essential as is assessing disease status to personalize recommendations. For example, EEN or CDED could be recommended for a patient with a low-risk phenotype whose goal is to reduce inflammation, whereas MD could be recommended as adjunctive therapy for a patient who wishes to improve general health or reduce symptoms. Finally, all patients can benefit from a discussion about nutrition, even if the recommendations are small steps toward healthy eating.

CLINICS CARE POINTS

- The incidence and prevalence of IBD is rising and this is likely secondary to environmental factors.
- There are epidemiologic associations between diet and the development of IBD and patients and their families believe that diet has an impact on disease course.
- There are diets that can be used as a treatment for patients with Crohn's disease because of their ability to heal the mucosa.
- There are other diets that can be used to improve symptoms in patients with IBD but which lack evidence for mucosal healing currently.

DISCLOSURES

Speakers Bureau for Abbott Nutrition. Consulting for Nestle Health Sciences.

REFERENCES

1. de Lange KM, Moutsianas L, Lee JC, et al. Genome-wide association study implicates immune activation of multiple integrin genes in inflammatory bowel disease. Nat Genet 2017;49:256–61.
2. Jostins L, Ripke S, Weersma RK, et al. Host-microbe interactions have shaped the genetic architecture of inflammatory bowel disease. Nature 2012;491:119–24.
3. Stalgis C, Deepak P, Mehandru S, et al. Rational combination therapy to overcome the plateau of drug efficacy in inflammatory bowel disease. Gastroenterology 2021;161:394–9.
4. Cosnes J, Gower-Rousseau C, Seksik P, et al. Epidemiology and natural history of inflammatory bowel diseases. Gastroenterology 2011;140:1785–94.
5. Ng SC, Shi HY, Hamidi N, et al. Worldwide incidence and prevalence of inflammatory bowel disease in the 21st century: a systematic review of population-based studies. Lancet 2018;390:2769–78.
6. Broussard JL, Devkota S. The changing microbial landscape of Western society: diet, dwellings and discordance. Mol Metab 2016;5:737–42.
7. Hou JK, Abraham B, El-Serag H. Dietary intake and risk of developing inflammatory bowel disease: a systematic review of the literature. Am J Gastroenterol 2011;106:563–73.
8. Ananthakrishnan AN, Khalili H, Konijeti GG, et al. A prospective study of long-term intake of dietary fiber and risk of Crohn's disease and ulcerative colitis. Gastroenterology 2013;145:970–7.
9. Lo CH, Lochhead P, Khalili H, et al. Dietary inflammatory potential and risk of Crohn's disease and ulcerative colitis. Gastroenterology 2020;159:873–883 e1.

10. Narula N, Wong ECL, Dehghan M, et al. Association of ultra-processed food intake with risk of inflammatory bowel disease: prospective cohort study. BMJ 2021;374:n1554.
11. Limdi JK, Aggarwal D, McLaughlin JT. Dietary practices and beliefs in patients with inflammatory bowel disease. Inflamm Bowel Dis 2016;22:164–70.
12. Cohen AB, Lee D, Long MD, et al. Dietary patterns and self-reported associations of diet with symptoms of inflammatory bowel disease. Dig Dis Sci 2013;58: 1322–8.
13. Zallot C, Quilliot D, Chevaux JB, et al. Dietary beliefs and behavior among inflammatory bowel disease patients. Inflamm Bowel Dis 2013;19:66–72.
14. Bramuzzo M, Grazian F, Grigoletto V, et al. Dietary beliefs in children and adolescents with inflammatory bowel disease and their parents. J Pediatr Gastroenterol Nutr 2022;75:e43–8.
15. Levine A, Rhodes JM, Lindsay JO, et al. Dietary guidance from the international organization for the study of inflammatory bowel diseases. Clin Gastroenterol Hepatol 2020;18:1381–92.
16. Miele E, Shamir R, Aloi M, et al. Nutrition in pediatric inflammatory bowel disease: a position paper on behalf of the porto inflammatory bowel disease group of the European society of pediatric gastroenterology, hepatology and nutrition. J Pediatr Gastroenterol Nutr 2018;66:687–708.
17. van Rheenen PF, Aloi M, Assa A, et al. The Medical Management of Paediatric Crohn's Disease: an ECCO-ESPGHAN Guideline Update. J Crohns Colitis 2020 Oct 7;jjaa161. https://doi.org/10.1093/ecco-jcc/jjaa161. Epub ahead of print. PMID: 33026087.
18. Swaminath A, Feathers A, Ananthakrishnan AN, et al. Systematic review with meta-analysis: enteral nutrition therapy for the induction of remission in paediatric Crohn's disease. Aliment Pharmacol Ther 2017;46:645–56.
19. Ungaro RC, Yzet C, Bossuyt P, et al. Deep remission at 1 year prevents progression of early Crohn's disease. Gastroenterology 2020;159:139–47.
20. Darr U, Khan N. Treat to target in inflammatory bowel disease: an updated review of literature. Curr Treat Options Gastroenterol 2017;15:116–25.
21. Borrelli O, Cordischi L, Cirulli M, et al. Polymeric diet alone versus corticosteroids in the treatment of active pediatric Crohn's disease: a randomized controlled open-label trial. Clin Gastroenterol Hepatol 2006;4:744–53.
22. Pigneur B, Lepage P, Mondot S, et al. Mucosal healing and bacterial composition in response to enteral nutrition vs steroid-based induction therapy-A randomised prospective clinical trial in children with Crohn's disease. J Crohns Colitis 2019; 13:846–55.
23. Connors J, Basseri S, Grant A, et al. Exclusive enteral nutrition therapy in paediatric Crohn's disease results in long-term avoidance of corticosteroids: results of a propensity-score matched cohort analysis. J Crohns Colitis 2017;11:1063–70.
24. Narula N, Dhillon A, Zhang D, et al. Enteral nutritional therapy for induction of remission in Crohn's disease. Cochrane Database Syst Rev 2018;4:CD000542.
25. Rubio A, Pigneur B, Garnier-Lengline H, et al. The efficacy of exclusive nutritional therapy in paediatric Crohn's disease, comparing fractionated oral vs. continuous enteral feeding. Aliment Pharmacol Ther 2011;33:1332–9.
26. Seidman EG. Nutritional management of inflammatory bowel disease. Gastroenterol Clin North Am 1989;18:129–55.
27. Afzal NA, Davies S, Paintin M, et al. Colonic Crohn's disease in children does not respond well to treatment with enteral nutrition if the ileum is not involved. Dig Dis Sci 2005;50:1471–5.

28. Buchanan E, Gaunt WW, Cardigan T, et al. The use of exclusive enteral nutrition for induction of remission in children with Crohn's disease demonstrates that disease phenotype does not influence clinical remission. Aliment Pharmacol Ther 2009;30:501–7.

29. Cuomo M, Carobbio A, Aloi M, et al. Induction of remission with exclusive enteral nutrition in children with Crohn's disease: determinants of higher adherence and response. Inflamm Bowel Dis 2022.

30. Sahu P, Kedia S, Vuyyuru SK, et al. Randomised clinical trial: exclusive enteral nutrition versus standard of care for acute severe ulcerative colitis. Aliment Pharmacol Ther 2021;53:568–76.

31. Gupta K, Noble A, Kachelries KE, et al. A novel enteral nutrition protocol for the treatment of pediatric Crohn's disease. Inflamm Bowel Dis 2013;19:1374–8.

32. Urlep D, Benedik E, Brecelj J, et al. Partial enteral nutrition induces clinical and endoscopic remission in active pediatric Crohn's disease: results of a prospective cohort study. Eur J Pediatr 2020;179:431–8.

33. Johnson T, Macdonald S, Hill SM, et al. Treatment of active Crohn's disease in children using partial enteral nutrition with liquid formula: a randomised controlled trial. Gut 2006;55:356–61.

34. Lee D, Baldassano RN, Otley AR, et al. Comparative effectiveness of nutritional and biological therapy in North American children with active Crohn's disease. Inflamm Bowel Dis 2015;21:1786 93.

35. Nguyen DL, Palmer LB, Nguyen ET, et al. Specialized enteral nutrition therapy in Crohn's disease patients on maintenance infliximab therapy: a meta-analysis. Therap Adv Gastroenterol 2015;8:168–75.

36. Britto S, Kellermayer R. Carbohydrate monotony as protection and treatment for inflammatory bowel disease. J Crohns Colitis 2019;13:942–8.

37. Van Den Bogaerde J, Cahill J, Emmanuel AV, et al. Gut mucosal response to food antigens in Crohn's disease. Aliment Pharmacol Ther 2002;16:1903–15.

38. Lionetti P, Callegari ML, Ferrari S, et al. Enteral nutrition and microflora in pediatric Crohn's disease. JPEN J Parenter Enteral Nutr 2005;29:S173–5 [discussion: S175-8], S184-S188.

39. Leach ST, Mitchell HM, Eng WR, et al. Sustained modulation of intestinal bacteria by exclusive enteral nutrition used to treat children with Crohn's disease. Aliment Pharmacol Ther 2008;28:724–33.

40. Dunn KA, Moore-Connors J, MacIntyre B, et al. Early changes in microbial community structure are associated with sustained remission after nutritional treatment of pediatric Crohn's disease. Inflamm Bowel Dis 2016;22:2853–62.

41. Fritsch J, Abreu MT. The microbiota and the immune response: what is the chicken and what is the egg? Gastrointest Endosc Clin N Am 2019;29:381–93.

42. Gatti S, Galeazzi T, Franceschini E, et al. Effects of the exclusive enteral nutrition on the microbiota profile of patients with Crohn's disease: a systematic review. Nutrients 2017;9.

43. Lewis JD, Chen EZ, Baldassano RN, et al. Inflammation, antibiotics, and diet as environmental stressors of the gut microbiome in pediatric Crohn's disease. Cell Host Microbe 2015;18:489–500.

44. Diederen K, Li JV, Donachie GE, et al. Exclusive enteral nutrition mediates gut microbial and metabolic changes that are associated with remission in children with Crohn's disease. Sci Rep 2020;10:18879.

45. Thomas AG, Taylor F, Miller V. Dietary intake and nutritional treatment in childhood Crohn's disease. J Pediatr Gastroenterol Nutr 1993;17:75–81.

46. Gerasimidis K, Talwar D, Duncan A, et al. Impact of exclusive enteral nutrition on body composition and circulating micronutrients in plasma and erythrocytes of children with active Crohn's disease. Inflamm Bowel Dis 2012;18:1672–81.

47. Newby EA, Sawczenko A, Thomas AG, et al. Interventions for growth failure in childhood Crohn's disease. Cochrane Database Syst Rev 2005;3:CD003873.

48. Whitten KE, Leach ST, Bohane TD, et al. Effect of exclusive enteral nutrition on bone turnover in children with Crohn's disease. J Gastroenterol 2010;45:399–405.

49. Guo Z, Wu R, Zhu W, et al. Effect of exclusive enteral nutrition on health-related quality of life for adults with active Crohn's disease. Nutr Clin Pract 2013;28: 499–505.

50. Afzal NA, Van Der Zaag-Loonen HJ, Arnaud-Battandier F, et al. Improvement in quality of life of children with acute Crohn's disease does not parallel mucosal healing after treatment with exclusive enteral nutrition. Aliment Pharmacol Ther 2004;20:167–72.

51. Svolos V, Gerasimidis K, Buchanan E, et al. Dietary treatment of Crohn's disease: perceptions of families with children treated by exclusive enteral nutrition, a questionnaire survey. BMC Gastroenterol 2017;17:14.

52. Sigall-Boneh R, Pfeffer-Gik T, Segal I, et al. Partial enteral nutrition with a Crohn's disease exclusion diet is effective for induction of remission in children and young adults with Crohn's disease. Inflamm Bowel Dis 2014;20:1353–60.

53. Levine A, Wine E, Assa A, et al. Crohn's disease exclusion diet plus partial enteral nutrition induces sustained remission in a randomized controlled trial. Gastroenterology 2019;157:440–450 e8.

54. Yanai H, Levine A, Hirsch A, et al. The Crohn's disease exclusion diet for induction and maintenance of remission in adults with mild-to-moderate Crohn's disease (CDED-AD): an open-label, pilot, randomised trial. Lancet Gastroenterol Hepatol 2022;7:49–59.

55. Sigall Boneh R, Van Limbergen J, Wine E, et al. Dietary therapies induce rapid response and remission in pediatric patients with active Crohn's disease. Clin Gastroenterol Hepatol 2021;19:752–9.

56. Szczubelek M, Pomorska K, Korolczyk-Kowalczyk M, et al. Effectiveness of Crohn's disease exclusion diet for induction of remission in Crohn's disease adult patients. Nutrients 2021;13.

57. Niseteo T, Sila S, Trivic I, et al. Modified Crohn's disease exclusion diet is equally effective as exclusive enteral nutrition: real-world data. Nutr Clin Pract 2022;37: 435–41.

58. Sigall Boneh R, Sarbagili Shabat C, Yanai H, et al. Dietary therapy with the Crohn's disease exclusion diet is a successful strategy for induction of remission in children and adults failing biological therapy. J Crohns Colitis 2017;11: 1205–12.

59. Scarallo L, Banci E, Pierattini V, et al. Crohn's disease exclusion diet in children with Crohn's disease: a case series. Curr Med Res Opin 2021;37:1115–20.

60. Verburgt CM, Dunn KA, Ghiboub M, et al. Successful dietary therapy in paediatric Crohn's disease is associated with shifts in bacterial dysbiosis and inflammatory metabotype towards healthy controls. J Crohns Colitis 2023;17:61–72.

61. Ghiboub M, Penny S, Verburgt CM, et al. Metabolome changes with diet-induced remission in pediatric Crohn's disease. Gastroenterology 2022;163:922–936 e15.

62. Ghiboub M, Boneh RS, Sovran B, et al. Sustained diet-induced remission in pediatric Crohn's disease is associated with kynurenine and serotonin pathways. Inflamm Bowel Dis 2023;29:684–94.

63. Svolos V, Hansen R, Nichols B, et al. Treatment of active Crohn's disease with an ordinary food-based diet that replicates exclusive enteral nutrition. Gastroenterology 2019;156:1354–1367 e6.
64. Gottschall E. Breaking the vicious cycle. kirkton. Ontario, Canada: The Kirkton Press; 1994.
65. Cohen SA, Gold BD, Oliva S, et al. Clinical and mucosal improvement with specific carbohydrate diet in pediatric Crohn disease. J Pediatr Gastroenterol Nutr 2014;59:516–21.
66. Obih C, Wahbeh G, Lee D, et al. Specific carbohydrate diet for pediatric inflammatory bowel disease in clinical practice within an academic IBD center. Nutrition 2016;32:418–25.
67. Suskind DL, Cohen SA, Brittnacher MJ, et al. Clinical and fecal microbial changes with diet therapy in active inflammatory bowel disease. J Clin Gastroenterol 2018; 52:155–63.
68. Suskind DL, Wahbeh G, Gregory N, et al. Nutritional therapy in pediatric Crohn disease: the specific carbohydrate diet. J Pediatr Gastroenterol Nutr 2014;58: 87–91.
69. Kaplan HC, Opipari-Arrigan L, Yang J, et al. Personalized research on diet in ulcerative colitis and Crohn's disease: a series of N-of-1 diet trials. Am J Gastroenterol 2022;117:902–17.
70. Lewis JD, Sandler RS, Brotherton C, et al. A randomized trial comparing the specific carbohydrate diet to a Mediterranean diet in adults with Crohn's disease. Gastroenterology 2021;161:837–852 e9.
71. Jowett SL, Seal CJ, Pearce MS, et al. Influence of dietary factors on the clinical course of ulcerative colitis: a prospective cohort study. Gut 2004;53:1479–84.
72. Sarbagili-Shabat C, Albenberg L, Van Limbergen J, et al. A novel UC exclusion diet and antibiotics for treatment of mild to moderate pediatric ulcerative colitis: a prospective open-label pilot study. Nutrients 2021;13.

When and Where Should Surgery Be Positioned in Pediatric Inflammatory Bowel Disease?

Aaron M. Lipskar, MD

KEYWORDS

- Surgery • Pediatric • Crohn disease (CD) • Ulcerative colitis (UC)

KEY POINTS

- Children and adolescents diagnosed with IBD often have more aggressive disease and surgery is an important part of the treatment options.
- Early consultation with a surgeon for children and adolescents with IBD is prudent to inform patients and their families before there is no other alternative.
- There is a large amount of heterogeneity among children and adolescents with IBD (especially CD) and the decision to include surgical options depends on the individual clinical situation and is best served by a multidisciplinary team.
- While operating on children and adolescents with CD is never curative but can help to improve symptoms, minimize corticosteroid use, allow for significant catch-up growth, and achieve clinical remission.
- The decision to operate in children and adolescents with colitis is based on refractory disease despite maximal medical management and the rare severe complications of the disease that mandate emergency surgery. The initial operation is most frequently a laparoscopic subtotal colectomy with end ileostomy with the eventual restoration of intestinal continuity after completion proctectomy and ileal pouch with anal anastomosis.

INTRODUCTION

Inflammatory bowel disease (IBD) is a spectrum of immune-dysregulated gastrointestinal (GI) disorders that creates mucosal inflammation of different parts of the intestinal tract and often leads to the end result of mucosal damage such as strictures, bleeding, fistulae, abscesses, and (rarely in the pediatric and adolescent population) dysplastic changes.[1]

Surgery and Pediatrics, Division of Pediatric Surgery, Cohen Children's Medical Center, Zucker School of Medicine at Hofstra/Northwell, 1111 Marcus Avenue, Suite M15, New Hyde Park, NY 11042, USA
E-mail address: alipskar@northwell.edu

Gastroenterol Clin N Am 52 (2023) 579–587
https://doi.org/10.1016/j.gtc.2023.06.001
0889-8553/23/© 2023 Elsevier Inc. All rights reserved.

gastro.theclinics.com

The incidence of IBD has steadily been on the rise in the pediatric and adolescent population, with almost 25% of patients being diagnosed before the age of 20 and many of those patients undergoing surgical interventions while still in that age group.[1,2] Two recent studies have reported data that for patients diagnosed with IBD under the age of 17, 24% of those with CD and 9% of those with UC will go on to require surgery during childhood.[3,4]

Historically, surgery has been considered the salvage treatment modality in IBD after patients are walked up a therapeutic ladder of medical therapy with their gastroenterologists. In that analogy, patients become progressively more deconditioned, and the surgical morbidity and disease recurrence was thought to be prohibitively high, leading to surgery being thought of as a "last-ditch" option for children and adolescents with IBD. In the modern era with the advent of newer treatment options (such as biologic therapy and precision medicine), this analogy is flawed, as patients are treated in a top-down model, often staying naïve to steroids and starting the highly effective newer therapies at diagnosis. Additionally, although the common teaching has been that a patient with CD that undergoes intestinal resection carries a 50% chance of needing another intestinal operation in their life, that statistic is based on pre-biologic and pre-precision medicine data. Future data may prove the actual incidence of needing repeat operations to be lower. These changes along with others to be discussed in this article have led to a necessary reconsideration of the role of surgery.

The goal of this article is to introduce when and where, and at times how, surgery should be positioned in pediatric and adolescent IBD. Many other excellent articles in the last 10 years have been published describing surgery in pediatric IBD as well as some clinical guidelines published as well.[5–15] Unlike those articles, rather than going through the various indications, surgical options, and perioperative considerations for surgery in children and adolescents with IBD, this article will instead discuss many of these issues in broader strokes with the underlying theme being the importance of individualized, multidisciplinary decision-making for this highly heterogenous group of patients.

DISCUSSION

IBD is generally differentiated into 2 main disease entities, Crohn disease (CD) and Ulcerative colitis (UC), with a third sub-entity of IBD-unclassified (IBD-U).[6] This is an overly simplistic model, as recent advances in the understanding and classification of IBD have demonstrated that there are many more phenotypes and subtypes of IBD, especially of CD. These include but are not limited to very early onset IBD (VEO-IBD), penetrating and/or stricturing small bowel and ileocolic CD, upper gastrointestinal CD, perianal CD, and Crohn colitis. And as CD can affect the entire GI tract from the mouth to the anus with skip lesions, some patients will have multiple of these subtypes.

While there are absolute indications for emergency surgery for both UC and CD, such as free perforation, complete bowel obstruction, and uncontrolled GI hemorrhage, these cases are the exception, and the majority of the time the decision to operate is made in a semi-urgent or semi-elective manner and is based on persistent symptoms from the end result of mucosal damage despite attempts at medical treatment. The most common presentations of disease for the surgeon taking care of children and adolescents with IBD are stricturing or penetrating ileocolic CD, perianal CD, and isolated colitis refractory to medical management. There are many other scenarios in pediatric and adolescent IBD that warrant surgical consideration, but for the sake of this discussion the focus will be on the above-mentioned indications.

Some of the important themes of the discussion surrounding the role of surgery in pediatric and adolescent IBD are as follows.

- Patients diagnosed with IBD in the pediatric age group often have more aggressive and extensive disease, and although newer treatment modalities may help more children and adolescents avoid surgery, many will still need consideration of surgical options as part of the treatment plan during their pediatric and adolescent periods.
- There is significant heterogeneity in the clinical presentation, clinical condition, and anatomic region affected in IBD, making it quite difficult to generate clear guidelines for the when and where of surgery that is applicable broadly. The decision to offer surgical interventions must be individualized, and patients and their families are best served by a multidisciplinary and multimodal approach.
- Some of the unique considerations in the pediatric and adolescent IBD populations when considering surgical options are psychosocial conditions, growth delay, and avoidance of long-term exposure to toxic therapies, especially corticosteroids.
- Early inclusion of a surgeon that has experience and expertise in pediatric and adolescent IBD as part of the multidisciplinary team, even when surgery is not clearly necessary at that time, is prudent and can lead to improvements in the patient's overall experience and the families' understanding the nuances of these often difficult decisions.

STRICTURING OR PENETRATING ILEOCOLIC AND SMALL BOWEL CROHN DISEASE

The initial description of CD has generally been credited to Drs. Crohn, Ginzburg, and Oppenheimer in their landmark article published in 1932 in the Journal of the American Medical Association entitled "Regional Ileitis: a pathologic and clinical entity."[16] In that article, the authors describe the full-thickness inflammation that is now well accepted in CD that leads to strictures, fistulae, and abscesses. What the authors got wrong was that the disease was isolated to the terminal ileum (TI) as we now know that CD can affect the entire GI system from the mouth to the anus.

Strategies for surgical intervention in children and adolescents with intestinal CD should adhere to the basic tenets of CD surgery, namely the concepts of preserving intestinal length, minimizing intraabdominal adhesions, and although surgery for CD is never curative, attempting to allow for clinical remission for limited disease burden.[8] Furthermore, special consideration should be given to children that have fallen off the growth curve, as early surgery performed before the growth plates have closed is quite effective in restoring growth.[8] Surgical interventions for severely symptomatic CD may also be beneficial in younger populations to avoid the adverse effects of long-term corticosteroids, and in fact many pediatric IBDologists aim to keep their pediatric CD patients steroid-naïve if possible.

Due to the heterogeneity of disease location and symptomatology, there is no "one size fits all" surgical algorithm for children and adolescents with CD.[7] When surgery is considered for intestinal CD, resection should generally be the goal, although stricturoplasty should be considered for long-segment disease that does not involve the terminal ileum. Despite the various and nuanced indications for surgery in children and adolescents with CD, the most common indication for intestinal surgical consideration remains structuring and/or penetrating ileal disease.

Surgical intervention for isolated short-segment terminal ileal disease that has led to end-result of mucosal damage, namely strictures, fistulae and/or abscesses, should at times be considered as an earlier rung in the therapeutic ladder rather than falling off of the ladder. For these patients, gastroenterologists may consider an attempt at medical therapy, but early consultation with a surgeon should be obtained. If a decision is made for surgical intervention, patients should be optimized from an infectious and nutritional perspective as best as possible. For isolated short-segment terminal ileal disease, the operation of choice should be a laparoscopic-assisted ileocolic resection with anastomosis if the surgeon is comfortable with minimally invasive techniques. Further perioperative considerations will be discussed later.

PERIANAL CROHN DISEASE

Perianal disease is quite common in pediatric and adolescent CD, ranging in incidence from 13% to 62%.[14] Additionally, perianal disease is often the presenting clinical finding in pediatric and adolescent CD. Clinically, perianal CD manifests as fissures, skin tags, and fistulae with or without associated perianal abscesses. In general, while fissures and skin tags can be painful and cosmetically disfiguring there are no specific surgical interventions indicated. In contrast, CD-related fistula-in-ano (FIA) and associated perianal abscesses can lead to severe pain and perineal sepsis. CD-related FIAs are often tortuous and complex as compared to idiopathic FIAs, and magnetic resonance imaging of the pelvis with intravenous contrast can be very helpful in allowing the treatment team to have a better understanding of the anatomy of the fistulae and the presence of undrained abscesses.

Nearly all patients with CD-related perianal abscesses and FIA will benefit from some degree of surgical intervention, although the more definitive procedures such as fistulotomy, mucosal advancement flap, ligation of the intersphincteric fistula tract (LIFT) procedure and fistula plug placement are rarely necessary due to the efficacy of biologic therapy when source control is accomplished. Most children and adolescents will benefit from an anorectal examination under anesthesia, drainage of perianal abscesses, and placement of non-cutting Setons in any identified fistulae. The role of the non-cutting Seton is simply to prevent ongoing abscess formation and to allow for the continuation or the initiation of proper medical therapy. Most recent guidelines have identified that the combination of anti-TNF therapy and source control with drainage and Setons are the treatment modality that allow for the best chance of healing and clinical remission.[13–15]

There are no clear data regarding when to remove Setons and the decision should be made by both the gastroenterologist and surgeon. One of the accepted approaches is to allow for the biologic therapy to reach a steady state (ex. after 3–4 infliximab infusions) and then remove the Seton if the perianal disease appears under control. At times follow-up MRIs are useful to better understand the burden of disease prior to Seton removal. Limited data exist for the use of endorectal ultrasound in the pediatric and adolescent population. There is little harm in leaving Setons for longer periods of time, as they are nearly always well tolerated.

Once the patient is in clinical remission, persistent FIAs without associated abscesses can be difficult to treat. Unless the FIA is found to be superficial and simple, formal fistulotomy should be avoided due to concerns for poor wound healing. Fistula plugs, LIFT procedure, and rectal mucosal advancement flaps have less issues with wound healing and have all been reported in the long-term management of CD-related FIA with varying success rates.[17] There are promising initial data regarding the efficacy of mesenchymal stem cells in pediatric and adolescent perianal CD although at the time of this publication access to this treatment modality in the pediatric population is limited.[18] Lastly, fecal diversion, while always an option for uncontrolled perineal sepsis, should only be considered in unique severe cases as these stomas can often end up being permanent as the recurrence rate after stoma reversal is reported to be well over 50%.[14]

Perianal CD in the pediatric population can be quite painful for children and can have a significant impact in patients' QOL. Like other surgical indications and decision-making processes in pediatric and adolescent CD, there is significant heterogeneity, and an individualized approach is necessary. Unlike with other clinical presentations of CD, nearly all patients with perianal abscesses and FIA will require some surgical intervention prior to initiating medical therapy, usually consisting of drainage of abscesses and placement of Setons. A multidisciplinary approach between surgeon and gastroenterologist is beneficial to provide the highest level of care for these patients.

ISOLATED COLITIS (USUALLY ULCERATIVE COLITIS) REFRACTORY TO MEDICAL MANAGEMENT

Colitis that is refractory to medical management is the most common indication for UC, and total proctolectomy is theoretically curative. Children and adolescents that do not respond well to medical management should meet with a surgeon experienced in UC as early as possible, as the procedures are complex, carry a high overall complication rate, and have long-term sequelae as far as quality of life.[10] Crohn colitis, especially segmental Crohn colitis, requires special consideration, as ileal pouches have significantly higher complication rates in the face of CD and recurrent disease after segmental resection is quite high.[8] Additional consideration needs to be given to the fact that a percentage of children and adolescents with UC will eventually be diagnosed with CD after total proctocolectomy.[19] Despite that, even with a diagnosis Crohn colitis, total proctocolectomy and ileal pouch creation should not be considered a contraindication, for as long as there is no active perianal or small bowel disease, as even though complications are more common, with proper treatment, pouch function can be acceptable and pouch failure rates remain reasonably low.[20]

For most children and adolescents with medically refractory colitis, a total abdominal colectomy with end ileostomy, leaving the rectum in place, should be considered the gold standard as the initial operation.[21] It carries a low complication rate and allows children to come off of all medications relatively quickly, achieve better nutritional status and improve dramatically from an emotional/psychological perspective, despite having an ileostomy. The decision on timing and method of future interventions should be based on surgeon experience, medical status of the patient, and patient/family understanding of the risks and benefits of the 3 main options: completion proctectomy with ileal pouch anal anastomosis with diverting loop ileostomy, undiverted completion proctectomy with ileal pouch anal anastomosis, and completion proctectomy with permanent ileostomy. An upfront total proctocolectomy with ileal pouch anal anastomosis with or without proximal diversion as an initial operation has become rare in patients with medically refractory disease due to the concerns for increased complications in the face of malnutrition, systemic inflammation, and medical therapies.

ADDITIONAL SURGICAL CONSIDERATIONS

Finally, it is important to briefly introduce some of the advances of the surgical approach that are becoming widely applicable and accepted in pediatric and adolescent IBD. These have led to improved outcomes and quicker recovery, allowing patients to resume or start additional medical therapies sooner after surgical interventions. Developments include but are not limited to the safety of surgery in patients being treated with biologic therapies, the liberal use of minimally invasive surgery, and the introduction of enhanced-recovery protocols in surgery for pediatric and adolescent IBD.

SURGERY AND BIOLOGIC THERAPIES

Despite early conflicting studies in both the adult and pediatric literature regarding the influence of biologic agents on postoperative complications, several studies in children and adolescents have not detected any difference in complications when comparing patients who did and did not receive biologic agents preoperatively.[22,23] It is generally now accepted that surgery should not be delayed in patients receiving biologic therapy, and in fact it may be detrimental for some patients to stop treatment in preparation for surgical intervention.

MINIMALLY INVASIVE SURGERY IN INFLAMMATORY BOWEL DISEASE

Since the advent of minimally invasive surgery (MIS) in the 1980s, laparoscopic techniques have evolved significantly and most recent graduates of general surgery programs in North America are trained and certified in advanced MIS. This has translated into MIS no longer being a subspecialty of general surgery but rather a technique that can be widely applied to many different operations. While there used to be a debate as to whether it would be better to have an MIS-trained or a colorectal-trained surgeon do laparoscopic colorectal surgery, this is no longer the case. For nearly all intraabdominal IBD operations, MIS has the advantage of decreased adhesion formation, improved cosmesis, and quicker recovery. Many operations for IBD involve a combination of MIS and open techniques, but most benefit significantly from some of the work being done laparoscopically.[8,10,24]

ENHANCED RECOVERY PROTOCOLS IN PEDIATRIC AND ADOLESCENT INFLAMMATORY BOWEL DISEASE

The goal of enhanced recovery protocols (ERPs) is to minimize the physiologic insult and stress of surgery and hasten recovery.[25] The basic concept is to institute various pre-, intra-, and postoperative elements such as perioperative patient education, limited fasting, euvolemic resuscitation, regional analgesia, MIS, avoidance of drains, early enteral intake, early postoperative mobilization, and limiting opioid utilization. ERPs have now been well established in the literature to lower length of stay, minimize narcotics, improve patient experience, and decrease complications.[25] ERPs were first developed and studied in adult colorectal surgery and have been slow to be adopted in pediatric surgery. Nevertheless, its usage in the pediatric and adolescent population is increasing, and pediatric and adolescent IBD surgery has been one of the areas where ERPs have been most widely applied and studied with similar results to the adult literature.[25]

SUMMARY

There is no question that despite the incredible advances in the understanding and medical treatment of pediatric and adolescent IBD, the surgeon continues to have an important role in these patients' care. This role has evolved along with advanced surgical techniques, novel medical therapies, and increasing data regarding the long-term outcomes. In pediatric and adolescent IBD, special consideration should be given to the fact that in the proper clinical scenario, earlier surgical intervention can improve patients' symptoms and emotional/psychological status, allow for significant catch-up growth, and avoid the adverse effects of many medical therapies, especially corticosteroids. Early consultation and involvement of a surgeon experienced in pediatric and adolescent IBD should always be the goal, as this allows for a multidisciplinary approach and can make the perioperative experience much less stressful for the patient and their families.

CLINICS CARE POINTS

- Children and adolescents diagnosed with IBD often have more aggressive disease and surgery is an important part of the treatment armamentarium.
- Early consultation with a surgeon for children and adolescents with IBD is prudent to inform patients and their families before there is no other option.
- There is a tremendous amount of heterogeneity among children and adolescents with IBD (especially CD) and the decision to include surgical options depends on the individual clinical situation and is best served by a multidisciplinary team.
- While operating on children and adolescents with CD is not curative it can help to improve symptoms, minimize corticosteroid use, allow for significant catch-up growth, and achieve clinical remission.
- The decision to operate in children and adolescents with colitis is based on refractory disease despite maximal medical management and the rare severe complications of the disease that mandate emergency surgery. The initial operation is most frequently a laparoscopic total abdominal colectomy with end ileostomy with the eventual restoration of intestinal continuity after completion proctectomy and ileal pouch with anal anastomosis.

DISCLOSURE

The author has nothing to disclose.

REFERENCES

1. Rosen MJ, Dhawan A, Saeed SA. Inflammatory Bowel Disease in Children and Adolescents. JAMA Pediatr 2015;169(11):1053–60.
2. Ye Y, Manne S, Treem WR, et al. Prevalence of Inflammatory Bowel Disease in Pediatric and Adult Populations: Recent Estimates From Large National Databases in the United States, 2007-2016. Inflamm Bowel Dis 2020;26(4): 619–25.
3. Blackburn SC, Wiskin AE, Barnes C, et al. Surgery for children with Crohn's disease: indications, complications and outcome. Arch Dis Child 2014;99(5): 420–6.
4. Ashton JJ, Versteegh HP, Batra A, et al. Colectomy in pediatric ulcerative colitis: A single center experience of indications, outcomes, and complications. J Pediatr Surg 2016;51(2):277–81.
5. Fuller MK. Pediatric Inflammatory Bowel Disease: Special Considerations. Surg Clin North Am 2019;99(6):1177–83.

6. Phillips MR, Brenner E, Purcell LN, et al. Pediatric Inflammatory Bowel Disease for General Surgeons. Surg Clin North Am. Kelay A, Tullie L, Stanton M. Surgery and paediatric inflammatory bowel disease. Transl Pediatr 2019;8(5):436–48.

7. Kim S. Surgery in Pediatric Crohn's Disease: Indications, Timing and Post-Operative Management. Pediatr Gastroenterol Hepatol Nutr 2017;20(1):14–21.

8. von Allmen D. Pediatric Crohn's Disease. Clin Colon Rectal Surg 2018; 31(2):80–8.

9. Amil-Dias J, Kolacek S, Turner D, et al. Surgical Management of Crohn Disease in Children: Guidelines From the Paediatric IBD Porto Group of ESPGHAN. J Pediatr Gastroenterol Nutr 2017;64(5):818–35.

10. Rentea RM, Renaud E, Ricca R, et al. Surgical Management of Ulcerative Colitis in Children and Adolescents: A Systematic Review from the APSA Outcomes and Evidence-Based Practice Committee [published online ahead of print, 2023 Feb 21]. J Pediatr Surg 2023;S0022-3468(23):00162-8.

11. Tan Tanny SP, Yoo M, Hutson JM, et al. Current surgical practice in pediatric ulcerative colitis: A systematic review. J Pediatr Surg 2019;54(7):1324–30.

12. Siow VS, Bhatt R, Mollen KP. Management of acute severe ulcerative colitis in children. Semin Pediatr Surg 2017;26(6):367–72.

13. de Zoeten EF, Pasternak BA, Mattei P, et al. Diagnosis and treatment of perianal Crohn disease: NASPGHAN clinical report and consensus statement. J Pediatr Gastroenterol Nutr 2013;57(3):401–12.

14. Forsdick VK, Tan Tanny SP, King SK. Medical and surgical management of pediatric perianal crohn's disease: A systematic review. J Pediatr Surg 2019;54(12): 2554–8.

15. Mutanen A, Pakarinen MP. Perianal Crohn's Disease in Children and Adolescents. Eur J Pediatr Surg 2020;30(5):395–400.

16. Crohn BB, Ginzburg L, Oppenheiner GD. Regional ileitis; a pathologic and clinical entity. Am J Med 1952;13(5):583–90.

17. Kantor N, Wayne C, Nasr A. What is the optimal surgical strategy for complex perianal fistulous disease in pediatric Crohn's disease? A systematic review. Pediatr Surg Int 2017;33(5):551–7.

18. Wang H, Jiang HY, Zhang YX, et al. Mesenchymal stem cells transplantation for perianal fistulas: a systematic review and meta-analysis of clinical trials. Stem Cell Res Ther 2023;14(1):103.

19. Fadel MG, Geropoulos G, Warren OJ, et al. Risks factors associated with the development of Crohn's disease after ileal pouch-anal anastomosis for ulcerative colitis: a systematic review and meta-analysis [published online ahead of print, 2023 Mar 24]. J Crohns Colitis 2023. https://doi.org/10.1093/ecco-jcc/jjad051. jjad051.

20. Lightner AL, Jia X, Zaghiyan K, et al. IPAA in Known Preoperative Crohn's Disease: A Systematic Review. Dis Colon Rectum 2021;64(3):355–64.

21. Denning NL, Kallis MP, Kvasnovsky CL, et al. Outcomes of Initial Subtotal Colectomy for Pediatric Inflammatory Bowel Disease. J Surg Res 2020;255:319–24.

22. Dotlačil V, Škába R, Roušková B, et al. Surgical treatment of Crohns disease in children in the era of biological treatment. Chirurgická léčba Crohnovy nemoci u dětí v éře biologické léčby. Rozhl Chir 2022;101(2):56–60.

23. Guo D, Jiang K, Hong J, et al. Association between vedolizumab and postoperative complications in IBD: a systematic review and meta-analysis. Int J Colorectal Dis 2021;36(10):2081–92.

24. Page AE, Sashittal SG, Chatzizacharias NA, et al. The role of laparoscopic surgery in the management of children and adolescents with inflammatory bowel disease. Medicine (Baltim) 2015;94(21):e874.
25. Vacek J, Davis T, Many BT, et al. A baseline assessment of enhanced recovery protocol implementation at pediatric surgery practices performing inflammatory bowel disease operations. J Pediatr Surg 2020;55(10):1996–2006.

The State of Clinical Trials in Pediatric Inflammatory Bowel Disease

Jeffrey S. Hyams, MD[a,b,*], Richard K. Russell, MD, PhD[c]

KEYWORDS

- Children • Inflammatory bowel disease • Crohn disease • Ulcerative colitis
- Clinical trials

KEY POINTS

- Children with inflammatory bowel disease (IBD) have far fewer treatment options than adults.
- Progress in extrapolating efficacy of adult clinical trials remains slow.
- Serious barriers remain to expediting advances in IBD treatment to children.

OVERVIEW

The increasing incidence and prevalence of inflammatory bowel disease (IBD) in children demonstrated during the past several decades[1–3] has underscored the importance of finding new and improved therapies for this population. Compared with adults, children with IBD often have more extensive disease, potential impairment of physical growth and sexual maturation, as well as significant psychosocial complications.[4,5] We emphasize from the start that clinical expression, disease pathogenesis, rates of disease complications, and response to therapy in children and adults are similar.[6–11] This is critical in ensuring that children have therapies that are as equally accessible as those for adults. Most importantly, children have the longest time horizon for IBD to affect their lives and yet this vulnerable population has historically *never* been at the forefront of new therapeutic discoveries, rather the opposite, with available therapies often becoming available only after many years following adult approval (**Table 1**).

[a] Division of Digestive Diseases, Hepatology, and Nutrition, Connecticut Children's Medical Center, 282 Washington Street, Hartford, CT 06106, USA; [b] University of Connecticut School of Medicine, Farmington, CT, USA; [c] Department of Paediatric Gastroenterology, Royal Hospital for Children and Young People, Clinical Staff Offices, 2nd Floor, 50 Little France Crescent, Edinburgh EH16 4TJ
* Corresponding author.
E-mail address: jhyams@connecticutchildrens.org

Gastroenterol Clin N Am 52 (2023) 589–597
https://doi.org/10.1016/j.gtc.2023.05.008
0889-8553/23/© 2023 Elsevier Inc. All rights reserved.

gastro.theclinics.com

Table 1
Gap between adult and pediatric approval of inflammatory bowel disease biologics and small molecules

Drug	Disease	Year Adult Approval	Year Pediatric Approval	Delay in Pediatric Approval
Infliximab	CD	1998	2006	8
Infliximab	UC	2005	2011	6
Adalimumab	CD	2008	2014	6
Adalimumab	UC	2012	2021	9
Certolizumab	CD	2008	*Not yet*	?
Golimumab	UC	2013	*Not yet*	?
Vedolizumab	CD	2014	*Not yet*	?
Vedolizumab	UC	2014	*Not yet*	?
Ustekinumab	CD	2016	*Not yet*	?
Ustekinumab	UC	2019	*Not yet*	?
Risankizumab	CD	2022	*Not yet*	?
Tofacitinib	UC	2018	*Not yet*	?
Upadacitinib	UC	2022	*Not yet*	?
Ozanimod	UC	2022	*Not yet*	?

Abbreviations: CD, Crohn disease; UC, ulcerative colitis.

The lack of timely regulatory approval for medications in children leads to their being labeled "experimental" by third-party payers who refuse to endorse their use without a laborious gantlet of time-consuming appeals.[12,13] These same payers demand failure of what has been termed "conventional" therapies (ie, corticosteroids, mesalamine, immunomodulators), which delays the start of more effective and generally safer medications. Indeed, biologic therapies and newer small molecules continue to be used earlier and earlier in children as they appear superior to older therapies for many patients.[14–16] Pediatric physicians are forced to resort to "off-label" use of biologics or small molecules based largely on adult studies before appropriate pharmacokinetic studies in children have been conducted. Historically, for many new drugs licensed in adults, the standard-of-evidence for pediatric use has become single center reports of experience (predominantly efficacy) with a limited number of patents.[17,18] Systematic safety reporting is nonexistent. Although attempts have been made to improve the process of extrapolation from adult studies to children, these attempts have continued to be incomplete and suboptimal. Although all will agree that dose and safety can never be extrapolated, there remains disagreement between regulators and industry as to whether efficacy can be extrapolated and to what extent. This article will explore the reasons for this historical and on-going unacceptable situation and offer potential pathways toward future improvement. A recent consensus meeting of relevant stakeholders emphasizes the important concepts reviewed in this article.[19]

CURRENT STATE

The number of high-quality randomized clinical trials within pediatric IBD to date is significantly limited. The prebiologic era was dominated largely by small poor-quality studies. There was often a lack of incentive/directives for pharmaceutical companies to perform appropriate studies in children, so they were simply not adequately done. There continues to be several difficulties and barriers to recruitment of adult patients with IBD to clinical trials, which all directly apply to pediatric IBD populations too. The situation is worse in pediatrics because the number of children with IBD is several fold less than adults, there are very few established large clinical research networks for pediatric trial coordination, and working with parents and families to take part in trials of new medications in children with active IBD is frequently difficult because of the historical insistence on placebo controlled trials.

The REACH study was the first biological licensing study to be carried out in children (n = 112, 34 centers over 1 year) with moderate/severe CD where patients were randomized after demonstrating initial response to 3 doses of infliximab into 1 of 2 maintenance dosing schedules (every 8 weeks vs 12 weeks).[9] This trial commenced several years after regulatory approval was given for infliximab in adults (1998) and culminated in pediatric licensing 8 years later (2006) highlighting the significant delay between pediatric and adult approval. That situation has not changed in the subsequent 16 years. Although vedolizumab was approved for adults with ulcerative colitis or Crohn disease in 2014, it has still not been approved for children. Golimumab (UC), certolizumab (CD), tofacitinib (UC), upadacitinib (UC), ustekinumab (CD, UC), risankizumab (CD), and ozanimod (UC) have all now been approved for adults. None is approved for children. The only biologics approved for children are infliximab and adalimumab.

Trying to simulate adult trials, regulatory authorities have historically mandated placebo-controlled arms in pediatric trials undermining the whole concept of extrapolation. Despite consistent and persistent advice from the pediatric IBD community that placebo-controlled trials were doomed to failure (ie, no enrollment), and frankly unethical, pharma and regulators pursued them anyway. Not surprisingly they were unsuccessful. This was exemplified by the precision crohn's disease management utilizing predictive protein panels (ENvISION) study, a placebo-controlled phase 3 randomized controlled study (RCT) of adalimumab in pediatric UC (NCT02065557). The initial study design had to be modified to remove randomization to placebo and change to use of an external placebo comparator after several years of minimal enrollment and expenditure of large amounts of money. Only after years of discussion did pharma and regulators realize that no parent of a child with active disease was going to allow their child to receive placebo instead of a medication that had *already been shown to be superior to placebo*.[20] These often heated discussions with the regulatory agencies eventually led to the belated recognition that placebo-controlled trials were not feasible for pediatrics.

CONTINUING BARRIERS TO CLINICAL TRIALS IN CHILDREN

Barriers to more timely study of emerging therapies and their introduction into the care of children with IBD continue to occur at multiple levels including industry, regulators, investigators, and patients/families. Safety, ethical, and financial concerns likely top the list of issues for industry with respect to starting pediatric studies.[21] There is great reluctance on the part of pharma to study children early in the development of a new drug because of the fear that any untoward event in a child might jeopardize adult trials and subsequent approval for adults. Industry thinks that adult approval might also be delayed if pediatric pK/pD studies were required before approval for adults. As the development of new therapies can cost billions of dollars, there exists a need to speed up the process and deliver adequate return to investors. Pediatric markets are considered small. The development of a pediatric investigational plan is a laborious and lengthy process with back-and-forth dialog that can continue for months to years. Pediatric trials are viewed as labor intensive, more costly per subject enrolled, and may require different formulation of an oral drug (liquid vs pill). There may be a simple cost–benefit analysis on the part of industry that suggests that pediatric trials should not occur until later in the life cycle of drugs marketed for adults.

Although the primary mission of regulatory bodies is to protect the welfare of clinical trial recipients, when taken to an extreme it can in fact delay the development of more effective and potentially safer therapies for children. An area of continued concern is the uncertainty of whether exposure–response is similar in adults and children and the degree to which extrapolation can be used. This issue was fully discussed in a recent article titled "Pediatric extrapolation of adult efficacy to children is critical for efficient and successful drug development."[22] The old maxim "you can never extrapolate dose or safety" for children is strongly endorsed by all those interested in drug development. This underscores the importance of establishing (when possible) solid exposure response data in adults with a range of doses that can then be used subsequently to examine pediatric dosing. Lack of these adult data delay the development of pediatric studies. Historically regulators have also insisted on study designs that they have been repeatedly advised are not feasible in children (long washout periods for previous drugs, extending corticosteroid exposure, placebo) and these studies have universally failed. In adult trials, a composite endpoint based on symptoms/patient reported outcome measures and endoscopy is desirable. However, regulators have insisted on similar endpoint measures in children including patient reported outcomes (PROs) that may be problematic in very young children and that do not yet exist. Delaying the study of a drug for lack of agreement on endpoints such as PROs continues to deprive children of access to newer therapies. In reality, the most important outcome, mucosal healing, is easy to standardize yet has not been adopted as a stand-alone outcome in many studies.

The performance of clinical trials is difficult for many pediatric clinicians who may not have adequate numbers of enrollable patients, suitable infrastructure to complete the time-consuming institutional review process, budgeting, and then actual performance of the trial. This is confounded by competing clinical activities that are deemed more immediate, lack of allocated time for research, and many centers lacking experience or training to take part in these often-complex studies. When the therapy to be studied is already approved in adults, clinicians may well opt to give the medication "off label" greatly simplifying the process and not having to abide by the strict rules (including dosing) of a clinical trial. The strict rules of clinical trial inclusion also mean that many children treated by clinicians would not be eligible for trial participation. However, if access to such a medication were only possible through a trial the decision-making process would be different for many clinicians.

There is also great concern over what we term "sham placebo." As pharma and regulators now recognize that placebo-controlled clinical trials of medications that have previously been shown in adults to be superior to placebo are unethical in children, there is often a "high dose" and "low dose" trial offered. In reality, the high dose is the dose found to be effective in adults and the low dose exactly that, a lower dose. In fact, for younger children if anything a higher dose may be needed making the use of a lower-than-adult equivalent dosing strategy less biologically plausible and bordering on unethical.[23] This was emphatically shown in the final pediatric trial of adalimumab for ulcerative colitis (ENVISION, NCT 02065557) where the final approved dose for maintenance was *higher* in children than in adults.

Knowing the importance of exposure response, clinicians are unwilling to accept what they consider may well be an inadequate dose. Most clinical trials enroll patients with moderate-to-severe disease who have failed multiple therapies. These patients are often on corticosteroids. Many clinical trials require that the steroid dose by held constant for 8 to 12 weeks, or until the earliest outcome determination. Although sound from a scientific standpoint, this practice does not mirror clinical practice where corticosteroids are tapered as soon as possible. Keeping an adolescent on 20 to 30 mg of prednisone daily for an additional 3 months is unacceptable. Finally, washout periods since the last dose of another biologic therapy may extend to 8 to 12 weeks. For patients with active disease, they simply cannot be held in limbo for this long while exhibiting moderate-to-severe symptoms. In clinical practice, new therapies are often started as soon as indicated without waiting for the previous therapy to be undetectable.

Patients and families are often reluctant to enter clinical trials because they fear being part of an "experiment." Paradoxically, they do not consider receiving the medication "off label" as experimental because it has already received regulatory approval, although in adults. It is common that once an IBD medication is approved in adults, the pediatric community rapidly explores its utility in children. The advantage for patients/families in using off-label versus clinical trial drug is a decreased burden of visits, likely less frequent blood draws, and perhaps fewer endoscopies. Yet, if the new medication is only available through a clinical trial, then the burden of these additional activities seems less to both patients/families and investigators. This is clearly demonstrated within pediatric trials in countries that do not have out-of-trial access to medications and subsequently have much higher recruitment than countries that do.[23] Without question, patients and families will not accept placebo-controlled trials of medications meant to be the primary therapy. Trials of medications that are "add ons" or ancillary therapy, may be more likely to be accepted even if placebo controlled.

A PATHWAY FORWARD
Accept Extrapolation of Efficacy from Adult Studies

The combination of too few enrollable pediatric patients and the community's unwillingness to utilize placebo-controlled comparator studies mandates acceptance that extrapolation of efficacy from adult studies is the only path forward. Until this is accepted, the situation in pediatric drug development will not significantly change. This tenet has been adopted in a PIBDnet consensus statement[24] as well as recent article from the practicing community and pharma.[22] The plethora of anti-tumor necrosis factor (anti-TNF) studies in adults and children provide adequate support for this.[25,26] Unfortunately, there are no clear regulatory mandates that will facilitate this approach. Indeed, the 2022 draft guidance documents issued by FDA on clinical trials in Crohn disease and ulcerative colitis do not even mention pediatric studies— (Crohn's disease. Ulcerative colitis. Developing drugs for treatment. Guidance for industry. April 2022.) U.S. Department of Health and Human Services, Food and Drug Administration, Center for Drug Evaluation and Research, Center for Biologics Evaluation and Research. It is critically important to develop adequate pharmacokinetic/pharmacodynamic data in young children (<30 kg) to ensure appropriate dosing.

Improve Study Design of Adult Studies to Support Subsequent/Parallel Pediatric Studies

Studies in adults need to focus beyond finding an adequate single dosing strategy that is better than placebo. Rather, there needs to be appropriate dose ranging/PK studies in adults that will eventually facilitate pediatric trials as well. This strategy could promote avoidance of a "low-dose" arm in pediatric trials and will reduce the number of patients needing to take part in the pediatric trial. It is important to remember that the dose approved by regulators is not necessarily the *best* dose. It is the dose that was used to compare with placebo and that was statistically significantly better. Pediatric dosing should seek to attain the ideal dose when possible. We have learned that lesson over and over with the widespread introduction of therapeutic drug monitoring.

Concurrent Recruitment of Children and Adults to Phase 3 Trials

The clear need for approval close in time to that in adults has already been discussed in detail. Recent studies of anti-interleukin 23 (anti-IL23) therapies have moved to reduce the minimum age of participants in some phase 3 study from 18 to 16 years. These were secondary add ons after the initial phase 3 trial had started with no specific recruitment target. This is an initial step in the right direction but a broader pediatric age group (12 years and older, minimum 40 kg weight) should be included from the outset of these phase 3 studies. There should be a priori agreement that these data can be used to support approval down to age of 12 years.

Decrease Patient Burden

Adopting trial designs that are more pragmatic and mirror clinical practice while still achieving meaningful clinical endpoints will reduce the burden on patients. This can be done for drugs caught in the hiatus between adult and pediatric approval. The Vedokids study is an example of how this can be done if concurrent approval has not been attained Vedokids was an investigator initiated study with prospectively collected pediatric data replacing the small case series or case reports that might have been done historically in the same adult to pediatric gap. Vedokids was prospective cohort of 142 patients that used no endoscopy but used clinical activity scores and the MINI index to examine rates of response and remission in children.[27] These studies compliment traditional clinical trial design and can be used to potentially reduce numbers or inform the pediatric licensing trial.

Platform Trials

Platform trials where different treatments can be assessed in parallel are a good potential option especially in pediatrics to maximize resources by sharing patients, investigators, and facilities within a single trial.[28] This should reduce the time needed for drug approval and aid logistical issues such as site set up where many pediatric sites are often needed to open for a small number of recruits per site. The downside of these studies is the increased logistics and complexity of getting agreement between companies to set up and then enact a master protocol. A pending platform trial will soon examine the utility of 2 p19 inhibitors, mirikizumab and guselkumab, in pediatric IBD.[28]

No Placebo

The reasons for this are obvious and already discussed but the principle, which has taken so long to be accepted, should remain enshrined as an essential feature of trial design moving forward.

Use Objective Endpoints

The lack of suitable PROs should not delay pediatric trials. Everyone can agree that endoscopic response and remission are objective and suitable endpoints. The pediatric community and patients/families are willing to utilize endoscopy at the start and finish of a suitable treatment period. If the proper duration of therapy to evaluate response is known from adult trials, then this would mean 2, not 3, procedures. A careful balance is needed especially if endoscopic healing data have been demonstrated in adults. Proxy assessments for mucosal healing such as the MINI index[29] can substitute for some endoscopic assessment perhaps most obviously in a trial postindication when the primary end point is at 52 weeks.

Safety Registries—Post Approval and Across Indications

A limited amount of safety information can be gathered within the course of an average pediatric clinical trial. Rare and serious complications can occur several years after license is granted so a postapproval registry looking for long-term complications across indications, not just limited to pediatric IBD, will help provide maximum information while not delaying access to the drug. The DEVELOP registry monitoring the long-term course of infliximab-treated patients can serve as an example of a successful platform.[30] The Pediatric IBD Foundation, ImproveCareNow, and the Critical Path Institute (C-Path) established the Children's Registry for the Advancement of Therapeutics (CREATE) in 2020. CREATE is a drug-agnostic safety registry designed facilitate postmarketing safety information. Such registries must be adequately funded to ensure investigator and patient participant commitment.

SUMMARY

It is unethical to fail to provide children with the same IBD therapies as adults. Industries that profit from the sale of therapeutics that are used in children with IBD, as well as regulatory agencies, have a moral and ethical imperative to reject the status quo, which delays their use.

DISCLOSURE

J.S. Hyams: Advisory Board Janssen, Lilly, Boehringer Ingelheim, Bristol Myers Squibb, consultant Takeda, United States, Pfizer, Abbvie. R.K. Russell—In the past 3 years, has received consultation fees, research grants, royalties, or honoraria from Janssen, United States, Pfizer, United States, AbbVie, United States, Takeda, Lilly, United States, Nestlé Health Science, United States, Pharmacosmos, and Celltrion, South Korea.

REFERENCES

1. Benchimol EI, Bernstein CN, Bitton A, et al. The Impact of Inflammatory Bowel Disease in Canada 2018: A Scientific Report from the Canadian Gastro-Intestinal Epidemiology Consortium to Crohn's and Colitis Canada. J Can Assoc Gastroenterol 2019;2:S1–5.

2. Ye Y, Manne S, Treem WR, et al. Prevalence of Inflammatory Bowel Disease in Pediatric and Adult Populations: Recent Estimates From Large National Databases in the United States, 2007-2016. Inflamm Bowel Dis 2020;26:619–25.

3. Ng SC, Shi HY, Hamidi N, et al. Worldwide incidence and prevalence of inflammatory bowel disease in the 21st century: a systematic review of population-based studies. Lancet 2017;390:2769–78.

4. Gower-Rousseau C, Dauchet L, Vernier-Massouille G, et al. The natural history of pediatric ulcerative colitis: a population-based cohort study. Am J Gastroenterol 2009;104:2080–8.

5. Brooks AJ, Rowse G, Ryder A, et al. Systematic review: psychological morbidity in young people with inflammatory bowel disease - risk factors and impacts. Aliment Pharmacol Ther 2016;44:3–15.

6. Van Limbergen J, Russell RK, Drummond HE, et al. Definition of phenotypic characteristics of childhood-onset inflammatory bowel disease. Gastroenterology 2008;135:1114–22.

7. Wang K, Zhang H, Kugathasan S, et al. Diverse genome-wide association studies associate the IL12/IL23 pathway with Crohn Disease. Am J Hum Genet 2009;84: 399–405.

8. Li K, Strauss R, Ouahed J, et al. Molecular Comparison of Adult and Pediatric Ulcerative Colitis Indicates Broad Similarity of Molecular Pathways in Disease Tissue. J Pediatr Gastroenterol Nutr 2018;67:45–52.

9. Hyams J, Crandall W, Kugathasan S, et al. Induction and maintenance infliximab therapy for the treatment of moderate-to-severe Crohn's disease in children. Gastroenterology 2007;132:863–73 [quiz: 1165–6].

10. Hyams J, Damaraju L, Blank M, et al. Induction and Maintenance Therapy with Infliximab for Children with Moderate-to-Severe Ulcerative Colitis. Clin Gastroenterol Hepatol 2012;10(4):391–9.e1.

11. Hyams JS, Griffiths A, Markowitz J, et al. Safety and efficacy of adalimumab for moderate to severe Crohn's disease in children. Gastroenterology 2012;143: 365–374 e2.

12. Constant BD, de Zoeten EF, Stahl MG, et al. Delays Related to Prior Authorization in Inflammatory Bowel Disease. Pediatrics 2022;149. e2021052501.

13. Kahn SA, Bousvaros A. Denials, Dilly-dallying, and Despair: Navigating the Insurance Labyrinth to Obtain Medically Necessary Medications for Pediatric Inflammatory Bowel Disease Patients. J Pediatr Gastroenterol Nutr 2022;75:418–22.

14. Sassine S, Zekhnine S, Qaddouri M, et al. Factors associated with time to clinical remission in pediatric luminal Crohn's disease: A retrospective cohort study. JGH Open 2021;5:1373–81.

15. Sassine S, Djani L, Cambron-Asselin C, et al. Risk Factors of Clinical Relapses in Pediatric Luminal Crohn's Disease: A Retrospective Cohort Study. Am J Gastroenterol 2022;117:637–46.

16. Walters TD, Kim MO, Denson LA, et al. Increased effectiveness of early therapy with anti-tumor necrosis factor-alpha vs an immunomodulator in children with Crohn's disease. Gastroenterology 2014;146:383–91.

17. Moore H, Dubes L, Fusillo S, et al. Tofacitinib Therapy in Children and Young Adults With Pediatric-onset Medically Refractory Inflammatory Bowel Disease. J Pediatr Gastroenterol Nutr 2021;73:e57–62.

18. Dayan JR, Dolinger M, Benkov K, et al. Real World Experience With Ustekinumab in Children and Young Adults at a Tertiary Care Pediatric Inflammatory Bowel Disease Center. J Pediatr Gastroenterol Nutr 2019;69:61–7.

19. Croft NM, de Ridder L, Griffiths AM, et al. Paediatric inflammatory bowel disease: a multi-stakeholder perspective to improve development of drugs for children and adolescents. J Crohns Colitis 2023;17(2):249–58.

20. Sandborn WJ, van Assche G, Reinisch W, et al. Adalimumab induces and maintains clinical remission in patients with moderate-to-severe ulcerative colitis. Gastroenterology 2012;142:257–65.e1-3.

21. Conroy S, McIntyre J, Choonara I, et al. Drug trials in children: problems and the way forward. Br J Clin Pharmacol 2000;49:93–7.

22. Mulberg AE, Conklin LS, Croft NM, et al. Pediatric Extrapolation of Adult Efficacy to Children Is Critical for Efficient and Successful Drug Development. Gastroenterology 2022;163:77–83.

23. Croft NM, Faubion WA Jr, Kugathasan S, et al. Efficacy and safety of adalimumab in paediatric patients with moderate-to-severe ulcerative colitis (ENVISION I): a

randomised, controlled, phase 3 study. Lancet Gastroenterol Hepatol 2021;6: 616–27.

24. Turner D, Griffiths AM, Wilson D, et al. Designing clinical trials in paediatric inflammatory bowel diseases: a PIBDnet commentary. Gut 2020;69:32–41.

25. Adedokun OJ, Xu Z, Padgett L, et al. Pharmacokinetics of infliximab in children with moderate-to-severe ulcerative colitis: results from a randomized, multicenter, open-label, phase 3 study. Inflamm Bowel Dis 2013;19:2753–62.

26. Sharma S, Eckert D, Hyams JS, et al. Pharmacokinetics and exposure-efficacy relationship of adalimumab in pediatric patients with moderate to severe Crohn's disease: results from a randomized, multicenter, phase-3 study. Inflamm Bowel Dis 2015;21:783–92.

27. Atia O, Shavit-Brunschwig Z, Mould DR, et al. Outcomes, dosing, and predictors of vedolizumab treatment in children with inflammatory bowel disease (VEDO-KIDS): a prospective, multicentre cohort study. Lancet Gastroenterol Hepatol 2023;8(1):31–42.

28. Nelson RM, Conklin LS, Komocsar WJ, et al. The Role of Master Protocols in Pediatric Drug Development. Ther Innov Regul Sci 2022;56:895–902.

29. Cozijnsen MA, Ben Shoham A, Kang B, et al. Development and Validation of the Mucosal Inflammation Noninvasive Index For Pediatric Crohn's Disease. Clin Gastroenterol Hepatol 2020;18:133–140 e1.

30. Hyams JS, Dubinsky MC, Baldassano RN, et al. Infliximab Is Not Associated With Increased Risk of Malignancy or Hemophagocytic Lymphohistiocytosis in Pediatric Patients With Inflammatory Bowel Disease. Gastroenterology 2017;152: 1901–19014 e3.

Building a Self-Management Toolkit for Patients with Pediatric Inflammatory Bowel Disease: Introducing the resilience 5

Sara Ahola Kohut, PhD[a],*, Laurie Keefer, PhD[b]

KEYWORDS

• IBD • Transition • Resilience • Adolescent • Young adult • Self-management

KEY POINTS

- Transition from pediatric to adult IBD healthcare is a complex process that calls for complex interventions and collaboration between healthcare teams and families.
- There are teachable skills that foster and support IBD self-management, offset disease interfering behaviors, and build resilience in young people with IBD.
- The Resilience5 skills (self-efficacy, disease acceptance, self-regulation, optimism, and social support) can be encouraged and reinforced during routine IBD clinical care.

The challenges of transitioning from pediatric to adult health care in the context of inflammatory bowel disease (IBD) are well documented from both patient and health care professional perspectives.[1–3] As rates of IBD rise and clinical teams take on larger patient loads, continuity of care and "warm handoffs" becomes increasingly difficult. To date, much of the focus in IBD care has remained in the areas of medications, surgical interventions, and nutritional management.[4] This often leaves patients and families to navigate the transition alongside the emotional ramifications of IBD.[5] Moreover, health care transitions occur at a developmental stage where one is simultaneously trying to become more independent and determine how to live a meaningful life with IBD. As such, psychological distress and rates of mental health disorders in IBD populations are high, in particular among young adults.[6–8] Early effective identification of psychological risk factors can lead to improved outcomes in both adolescent and adult IBD populations.[9]

[a] Department of Gastroenterology, Hepatology, and Nutrition, Hospital for Sick Children, 555 University Avenue, Toronto, Onatrio, Canada; [b] Icahn School of Medicine at Mount Sinai, 1 Gustave L. Levy Place, New York, NY, USA
* Corresponding author.
E-mail address: sara.aholakohut@sickkkids.ca

Gastroenterol Clin N Am 52 (2023) 599–608
https://doi.org/10.1016/j.gtc.2023.05.005
0889-8553/23/© 2023 Elsevier Inc. All rights reserved.

Several approaches to transition have been explored in the literature with challenges to maintaining robust transition supports in routine clinical care.[6,10,11] Research supports several core components in encouraging successful transitions from pediatric to adult health care such as appropriate assessment, disease-related education, skill building, and communication and collaboration between families and their pediatric and adult health care teams (**Table 1**).[12–14] In the absence of resources to implement a robust transition program, clinical teams may refer to these components to identify ways to encourage successful transitions. With respect to assessment, many disease self-management and transition measures as well as indicators of transition success currently exist to help identify gaps in knowledge and skill in adolescent and young adult patients.[15,16] However, there are no current gold standard measures specific to the IBD transition process.[17] Clinical teams must consider feasibility of implementing both the assessment measures and addressing any needs that are identified through the assessment process. Similarly, IBD education materials also currently exist and are freely available through local and national foundations (eg, Crohn's and Colitis Foundation of America, Crohn's and Colitis Canada) as well as health care institutions. However, families have identified it is essential that IBD clinical teams support them by communicating and providing information on accessing accurate education.[18] Thus, assessing patients and families' needs and providing them with appropriate educational materials are necessary first steps in supporting disease self-management and encouraging successful health care transition.

Table 1
Core components in encouraging successful transitions from pediatric to adult healthcare

Core Component	Description
Individualized assessment	Biopsychosocial risk profile as determined via the following domains: • Quality of life (biological, psychological, social, family, health system) • Self-efficacy • Functioning • Transition readiness • IBD knowledge
Education	Structured eLearning curriculum focused on: • Healthy lifestyle • Transitioning to adult care • Self-care • Practical approaches to IBD-related tasks • Knowledge of IBD (eg, disease location, medications)
Skill building	Skill building in the domain of resilience, with particular focus on: • Assertiveness, self-regulation, IBD-related self-efficacy • Skill building in Resilience5 skills Navigating insurance and costs of IBD care Knowledge of pharmacy and obtaining medications Additional skill building as determined by patient navigator
Collaboration	Patient navigator (ie, nurse, nurse practitioner, or social worker) that follows across both settings and has understanding of IBD *Note*: in the absence of patient navigators, transition facilitation can be accomplished via collaboration between pediatric and adult health care teams

For full protocol see: Bollegala N, Barwick M, Fu N, et al. Multimodal intervention to improve the transition of patients with inflammatory bowel disease from pediatric to adult care: protocol for a randomized controlled trial. BMC Gastroenterology. 2022;22(1):1–13.

In addition to assessment and education, there are skills that can be acquired that support quality of life and mental health in young people with IBD. Moreover, these skills can simultaneously target disease-interfering self-management behaviors. Disease-interfering self-management behaviors (eg, catastrophizing or fear of pain, pessimism, psychological inflexibility, low self-confidence, and low social support) are well documented in the literature to be related to poor outcomes in young people with IBD.[19–21] However, these disease-interfering behaviors also provide the earliest window of opportunity to address the link between mental health and IBD outcomes. These behaviors may be the result of the patient, their family, the health care team/ professional, or the patient's environment that impede optimal medical and/or surgical outcomes in patients living with IBD. Addressing disease interfering behaviors allows for a unique opportunity to engage in preventative care and build capacity for navigating life with IBD.

Although appropriate assessment and IBD education approaches currently exist,[2] less is known and readily available with respect to targetable skills to support resilience and health care transitions. Given the current barriers to accessing robust transition programs in IBD clinical settings, clinical teams must adopt interventions that are readily accessible in routine clinical care. This review presents a model of skills that can be fostered at multiple clinical care points that support disease self-management, successful transition to adult health care, and overall mental health and well-being. This model can be used to foster resilience and also to identify and remediate deficits in the skills that encourage positive adaptation to living with IBD.

RESILIENCE5 MODEL

An approach developed and validated by Keefer and colleagues[22] highlights 5 core components that prevent disease interfering self-management behaviors, known as the Resilience5: self-efficacy, disease acceptance, self-regulation, optimism, and social support. The Resilience5 model (**Fig. 1**) is transdiagnostic across all chronic conditions and can be personalized to reflect disease specific self-management behaviors. Moreover, the Resilience5 can be applied to either a single outcome of interest (eg, medication adherence) or to several outcomes at once (eg, medication adherence and quality of life). Conversely, each individual component of the Resilience5 can be assessed and learned individually or as a whole. The flexibility of this model allows for the care team to identify patient needs and motivations to support overall well-being. Many skills can be fostered and reinforced during routine clinical appointments and do not require lengthy explanations or conversations. The components of the Resilience5 are also interconnected in that supporting the development and skill acquisition in one component supports skill acquisition in all other components.

Self-Efficacy

Self-efficacy is one's self-confidence and belief in one's ability to engage in and complete a task or goal. In the context of IBD, this often relates to one's self-confidence in following the recommended treatment plan. However, IBD self-efficacy also includes the self-confidence that, although one may not have total control of symptoms, they can work with what they can control and be successful.[23] Self-efficacy and self-confidence have been shown to predict behavioral intention and follow-through. In fact, self-efficacy and resilience scores predicted over 50% of transition readiness scores in a sample of adolescents and young adults with IBD.[24] Self-efficacy can be fostered in clinical settings via health care professionals by the language used

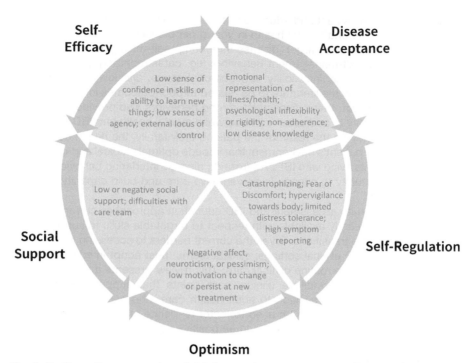

Fig. 1. Resilience5 components and risk factors they can prevent and/or remediate.

with patients. For example, health care team members can share confidence in their patient's ability to navigate fear and anxiety versus "do not be afraid" or share their confidence in their patient's ability to adhere to medications and undergo procedures. Supporting disease self-efficacy can also be accomplished by highlighting or noting other areas of success in a patient's life (eg, graduation, acceptance into postsecondary education, obtaining employment, or success in hobbies or valued activities).

Disease Acceptance

Disease acceptance is an active process whereby one aims to acknowledge and work with the realities of inevitable IBD symptoms and treatment. Acceptance is not about being resigned but instead about a willingness to work with IBD in service of living a valued and meaningful life. For example, accepting the uncertainty of IBD flares while remaining engaged in day-to-day activities or responsibilities that matter to you. Acceptance can help youth determine when their symptoms require them to rest versus "push through" and can improve self-efficacy and fatigue. Disease acceptance is also a key feature in one's ability to be psychologically flexible and work with unavoidable disappointments or setbacks of life. Avoidance-based approaches are particularly problematic in IBD and impact transition readiness by preventing the ability to learn how to cope and navigate the physical, emotional and social outcomes associated with IBD. Avoidance or safety-based behaviours can also indicate mental health or socio-economic concerns that warrant referral to mental health professionals or social services. For a sample of acceptance versus avoidance-based behaviors to help care teams identify risk factors and possible points in intervention (**Fig. 2**).

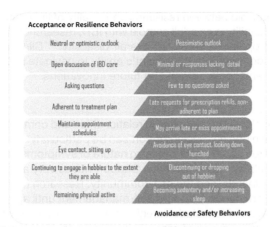

Fig. 2. Examples of acceptance and avoidance-based behaviors seen in clinic.

Self-Regulation

Self-regulatory skills include strategies that allow the individual to manage uncomfortable or unpleasant thoughts, feelings, behaviors, or impulses in pursuit of a short or long-term goal. Emotional self-regulation is perhaps the most challenging—adolescents with chronic illnesses must learn to attend to versus remove negative emotions, and use them instead to inform their behavior to reach their goals. Adolescents and young adults who can self-regulate have better educational and ultimately career trajectories, social skills and relationships and overall better health.[25] There are several self-regulatory challenges in the management of IBD, including tolerating unpredictable bowel symptoms, fatigue or pain, undergoing invasive procedures, self-injections, navigating complex medical and pharmacy benefits plans, managing frustration associated with delays in care, and having to remain organized with respect to routine labs, vaccines and surveillance recommendations. Self-regulation around the shifting responsibility of disease self-management tasks from caregivers to the adolescent emerged as an important transition readiness skill in a study that used photovoice methodology.[3] Clinical teams can encourage young people to engage in self-care behaviors and coping strategies, in particular with the goal of curating a personalized list of self-regulatory techniques.

Optimism

Optimism is about adopting a hopeful outlook on the future. Often this involves remaining open and having confidence while acknowledging the uncertainty of the future. We often encourage adolescents to focus on the "3 Ps" of optimism; viewing the cause of positive events as *Personal, Permanent,* and *Pervasive* and the cause of negative events (an IBD diagnosis or flare, a surgery, or set-back) as the opposite; not personal, as temporary, and as an isolated experience (vs. all-encompassing).[26] Optimism in this context, and alongside disease acceptance, is also differentiated from other maladaptive forms of positivity in which an individual feels they must always focus on only positive aspects and mindsets while ignoring all struggle or negative or unwanted feelings or experiences. Although less researched than other components of the Resilience5, optimism is helpful in maintaining motivation to engage in disease self-management as well as to persevere through flare-ups and IBD set-backs. Moreover, a small cross-sectional study of adolescents living with IBD found that optimism mediated the relationship between resilience and quality of life relative to IBD.[27] Similarly, in a study of disability in an adult sample with IBD, researchers found that gender, comorbidities, and optimism predicted overall disability.[28] Clinical care teams can offer optimistic outlooks on both the patient's ability to navigate IBD and/or their optimism in IBD treatments, both current and future innovations.

Social Support

Social support is one's ability to engage in relationships and community to aid in overall health care and well-being. Social support can be particularly challenging in the IBD context given the often socially embarrassing nature of symptoms, dietary restrictions, and potential unreliability due to IBD flare. Support needs vary and can be accessed via family, partners, friends, and the IBD community. Research has shown youth with IBD do not master independent disease self-management until age 21 years or older, thus highlighting the need to include caregivers in the transition process.[29] However, there is also a need to be aware of caregiver behaviors that help and hinder independent IBD self-management. For example, caregiver miscarried helping has been found to be related to increased adolescent reported pain in IBD.[30] Conversely, being engaged in the IBD community has also been shown to support transitional aged youth's overall well-being.[3,23,31] For caregiving behaviors related to IBD self-management and sample interventions that can be implemented in routine clinical practice (**Fig. 3**).

In addition to social support via family and community, young people with IBD benefit from active engagement and collaboration with their health care teams. Health care teams and caregivers may begin to engage in fostering resilience in young people with IBD at any age (See **Table 2** for examples of behaviors that support resilience building in others via the Resilience5). To the extent possible, it is also beneficial for pediatric and adult IBD clinical care teams to collaborate to support transition versus transfer of care.[32] Implementation of the Resilience5 via patient navigators is currently being studied in Canada to support the transition from pediatric to adult health care (please see open access Bollegala and colleagues, 2022 for study protocol).[12] This study is actively exploring a multimodal intervention that, after specialized

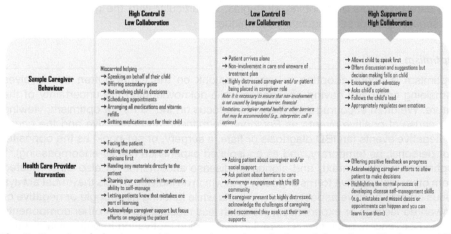

Fig. 3. Caregiver behaviors and intervention points. (*Adapted from* Levy, Keefer, van Tilburg, 2017).

Table 2
Tips to encourage Resilience5 skills in clinic

Resilience5 Skill	Health Care Team and Caregiver Tips
Self-efficacy	• Highlighting for patients what they are doing well • Providing positive feedback for effort and not outcome • Being mindful with language around success/failure or treatment and outcomes (eg, saying a medication failed vs the patient failed a medication) • Recommending and/or offering assertiveness training
Disease acceptance	• Offering IBD education and clear care plan • Acknowledging efforts at remaining engaged in life • Validating the frustrations of living with uncertainty while highlighting other patients similar lived experience • Encouraging flexible approach to living with IBD while aiming for remission vs trying to have total control over all symptoms
Self-regulation	• Offering mental health education and supports making referrals as necessary • Encouraging learning and engaging in coping skills, mindfulness, relaxation exercise and gut-directed hypnosis • Noting when patients successfully engage in adaptive coping • Validating emotional concerns and emotional aspects of IBD
Optimism	• Having an optimistic outlook on the patient's ability and capacity to learn and cope • Asking patients and families what is going well, what is going right? • Focusing on what patients and families were able to accomplish despite symptoms or setbacks • Sharing optimism in new treatments and approaches to living with IBD
Social support	• Inviting patients and families to engage in the IBD community • Involving patients and families actively in research as patients partners • Active listening and collaborating by allowing space for patients and families to ask questions and make informed decisions • If needed, refer for social skills training • If caregiver distress is present, encourage them to obtain their own mental health or social support

assessment, includes the combination of IBD education, resilience skill building, and patient navigators in supporting adolescents and young adults with IBD.

Transition to adult health care is a complex process that demands complex and multidimensional solutions. However, not all centers or clinics have the capacity to engage in additional complex interventions. The approaches highlighted in this review aim to offer clinical care teams readily implementable strategies to begin to engage and reinforce health behaviors that encourage successful transitions. In addition, a recent review describes how clinical care teams can adopt a psychogastroenterology perspective on transitions and outlines 5 patient-centered interventions that can also be implemented in the context of routine clinical care (see open access Mendiolaza and colleagues 2022).[1] Taken together, although health care transitions are a challenging time for both patients, their families, and health care professionals; there are readily available and teachable skills that will increase resilience in young people with IBD.

SUMMARY

Adolescence and young adulthood are challenging developmental periods with many transitions (eg, to postsecondary education, to occupations, to independent living) unrelated to the health care transitions in IBD populations. These young people are at increased risk of poor health care transitions and disease self-management. Although comprehensive IBD care is not readily available in all areas and centers, this review offers a list of skills and behaviors that can be encouraged in everyday clinical practice to support resilience in patients and families. Multimodal care, as described in this review, will support successful health care transitions and IBD disease self-management in adolescents and young adults with IBD.

CLINICS CARE POINTS

- In service of supporting successful transition from pediatric to adult healthcare, health care professionals and teams are encouraged to implement the following approaches to the extent in which they are able in their clinics.
- Individualized assessments of biopsychosocial risk (exploring biological, psychological, social, family and health systems), IBD disease knowledge and self-management, and transition readiness. This includes identifying what support may be needed during and after transfer to adult IBD care.
- Provide or help patients access evidence based multidisciplinary IBD education (e.g., knowledge and understanding of IBD and IBD treatments, IBD self-management, healthy lifestyle, self-care techniques).
- Encourage and reinforce the development of skills needed for successful transitions including Resilience5 skills (see Table 2 for approaches that can be implemented during routine IBD clinic appointments) as well as day to day self-management (e.g., calling in prescription refills, awareness of insurance guidelines, when to call for an appointment etc...)
- Collaboration between the pediatric and adult IBD healthcare teams. This includes ensuring a comprehensive and timely transfer of documents and medical history, results of the individualized assessment to help highlight areas of youth and family needs, and when possible, meetings or joint pediatric and adult IBD clinic appointments.

DISCLOSURE

S. Ahola Kohut: Joint copyright owner iPeer2Peer Peer Mentor Training. L. Keefer: equity owner, consultant Trellus Health.

REFERENCES

1. Mendiolaza ML, Feingold JH, Kaye-Kauderer HP, et al. Transitions from pediatric to adult IBD care: Incorporating lessons from psychogastroenterology. Frontiers in Gastroenterology 2022;1:1037421. https://doi.org/10.3389/fgstr.2022.1037421.
2. Rohatinsky N, Risling T, Kumaran M, et al. Healthcare transition in pediatrics and young adults with inflammatory bowel disease. Gastroenterol Nurs 2018;41(2):145–58.
3. Feingold JH, Kaye-Kauderer H, Mendiolaza M, et al. Empowered transitions: Understanding the experience of transitioning from pediatric to adult care among adolescents with inflammatory bowel disease and their parents using photovoice. J Psychosom Res 2021;143:110400.
4. Rutgeerts P, Vermeire S, Van Assche G. Mucosal healing in inflammatory bowel disease: impossible ideal or therapeutic target? Gut 2007;56(4):453–5.
5. Keefer L. and Kane S., Self-management techniques in IBD, In: Cross R., Watson A., (eds) Telemanagement of inflammatory bowel disease, 2016, Springer, Cham, 55–70. https://doi.org/10.1007/978-3-319-22285-1_5.

6. Volpato E, Bosio C, Previtali E, et al. The evolution of IBD perceived engagement and care needs across the life-cycle: a scoping review. BMC Gastroenterol 2021; 21(1):1–17.

7. Reigada LC, Bruzzese JM, Benkov KJ, et al. Illness-specific anxiety: Implications for functioning and utilization of medical services in adolescents with inflammatory bowel disease. J Spec Pediatr Nurs (JSPN) 2011;16(3):207–15.

8. Greenley RN, Hommel KA, Nebel J, et al. A meta-analytic review of the psychosocial adjustment of youth with inflammatory bowel disease. J Pediatr Psychol 2010;35(8):857–69.

9. Weaver E, Szigethy E. Managing pain and psychosocial care in IBD: a primer for the practicing gastroenterologist. Curr Gastroenterol Rep 2020;22(4):1–12.

10. Bollegala N, Nguyen GC. Transitioning the adolescent with IBD from pediatric to adult care: a review of the literature. Gastroenterology Research and Practice 2015;2015. https://doi.org/10.1155/2015/853530.

11. Abraham BP, Kahn SA. Transition of care in inflammatory bowel disease. Gastroenterol Hepatol 2014;10(10):633.

12. Bollegala N, Barwick M, Fu N, et al. Multimodal intervention to improve the transition of patients with inflammatory bowel disease from pediatric to adult care: protocol for a randomized controlled trial. BMC Gastroenterol 2022;22(1):1–13.

13. Kumagai H, Suzuki Y, Shimizu T. Transitional care for patients with inflammatory bowel disease: Japanese experience. Digestion 2021;102(1):18–24.

14. Kumagai H, Shimizu T, Iwama I, et al. A consensus statement on health-care transition for childhood-onset inflammatory bowel disease patients. Pediatr Int 2022; 64(1):e15241.

15. Kim J, Ye BD. Successful transition from pediatric to adult care in inflammatory bowel disease: what is the key? Pediatric Gastroenterology, Hepatology & Nutrition 2019;22(1):28–40.

16. Stinson J, Kohut SA, Spiegel L, et al. A systematic review of transition readiness and transfer satisfaction measures for adolescents with chronic illness. Int J Adolesc Med Health 2014;26(2):159–74.

17. Bihari A, Olayinka L, Kroeker KI. Outcomes in Patients with Inflammatory Bowel Disease Transitioning from Pediatric to Adult Care: A Scoping Review. J Pediatr Gastroenterol Nutr 2022;75(4):423–30.

18. Hait E, Arnold JH, Fishman LN. Educate, communicate, anticipate—practical recommendations for transitioning adolescents with IBD to adult health care. Inflamm Bowel Dis 2006;12(1):70–3.

19. Wojtowicz AA, Greenley RN, Gumidyala AP, et al. Pain severity and pain catastrophizing predict functional disability in youth with inflammatory bowel disease. Journal of Crohn's and Colitis 2014;8(9):1118–24.

20. Mackner LM, Crandall WV. Long-term psychosocial outcomes reported by children and adolescents with inflammatory bowel disease. Journal of the American College of Gastroenterology| ACG 2005;100(6):1386–92.

21. Kamp KJ, West P, Holmstrom A, et al. Systematic review of social support on psychological symptoms and self-management behaviors among adults with inflammatory bowel disease. J Nurs Scholarsh 2019;51(4):380–9.

22. Keefer L, Gorbenko K, Siganporia T, et al. Resilience-based integrated IBD care is associated with reductions in health care use and opioids. Clin Gastroenterol Hepatol 2022;20(8):1831–8.

23. Ahola Kohut S, Forgeron P, McMurtry M, et al. Resilience Factors in Paediatric Inflammatory Bowel Disease: Health Care Provider, Parent and Youth Perspectives. J Child Fam Stud 2021;30(9):2250–63.

24. Carlsen K, Haddad N, Gordon J, et al. Self-efficacy and resilience are useful pre-dictors of transition readiness scores in adolescents with inflammatory bowel dis-eases. Inflamm Bowel Dis 2017;23(3):341–6.
25. Keefer L. Behavioural medicine and gastrointestinal disorders: the promise of positive psychology. Nat Rev Gastroenterol Hepatol 2018;15(6):378–86.
26. Seligman ME, Steen TA, Park N, et al. Positive psychology progress: empirical validation of interventions. Am Psychol 2005;60(5):410.
27. Hare C, McMurtry M, Forgeron P, et al. Exploring the role of resilience in promot-ing health-related quality of life in adolescents with inflammatory bowel disease: The role of optimism and mindfulness. (in preparation).
28. Costa JM, Matos D, Arroja B, et al. The main determinants of disability in IBD and its relationship to optimism. Revista Espanola de Enfermadades Digestivas (REED) 2019;111(8):579–86.
29. Stollon N, Zhong Y, Ferris M, et al. Chronological age when healthcare transition skills are mastered in adolescents/young adults with inflammatory bowel disease. World J Gastroenterol 2017;23(18):3349.
30. Murphy LK, Rights JD, Ricciuto A, et al. Biopsychosocial correlates of presence and intensity of pain in adolescents with inflammatory bowel disease. Frontiers in Pediatrics 2020;8:559.
31. Ahola Kohut S, Stinson J, Jelen A, et al. Feasibility and acceptability of a mindfulness-based group intervention for adolescents with inflammatory bowel disease. J Clin Psychol Med Settings 2020;27(1):68–78.
32. Dabadie A, Troadec F, Heresbach D, et al. Transition of patients with inflammatory bowel disease from pediatric to adult care. Gastroenterol Clin Biol 2008;32(5): 451–9.

Health Care Maintenance in Pediatric Inflammatory Bowel Disease

Elana B. Mitchel, MD, MSCE*, Andrew Grossman, MD

KEYWORDS

- Pediatric inflammatory bowel disease • Health care maintenance • Preventative care
- Screening • Immunization • Malignancy

KEY POINTS

- Patients with pediatric inflammatory bowel disease (pIBD) are at an increased risk for complications and comorbidities because of both chronic systemic inflammation and exposure to immunosuppressive therapies.
- Complications and comorbidities that can develop include infection, nutritional deficiencies, growth and/or pubertal delay, bone disease, eye disease, malignancy, and psychologic issues.
- Preventative health maintenance with monitoring is important, although practice in pIBD is variable with limited data and guidelines.
- A multidisciplinary team with close work between the gastroenterologist provider and primary care provider is essential to successful health maintenance.

INTRODUCTION

Twenty five percent of patients with inflammatory bowel disease (IBD) or pIBD will be diagnosed by 18 years of age and classified.[1,2] The incidence of pIBD is increasing in North America with an estimated prevalence of 77 per 100,000 in 2016.[3,4] Pediatric-onset IBD poses unique challenges because it is often more extensive with a more aggressive disease course and requires greater immunosuppression as compared with adult-onset IBD.[5–8] Therefore, patients with pIBD are at an increased risk for developing complications and comorbidities both because of chronic systemic inflammation and the immunosuppressive therapies used.[9,10]

Complications and comorbidities include infection, nutritional deficiencies, growth delay and failure, bone disease, eye disease, malignancy, and psychologic disorders.[9,11] Many of these issues are avoidable and thus incorporation of preventative

Children's Hospital of Philadelphia, Gastroenterology, Hepatology and Nutrition, 3500 Civic Center Boulevard, Floor 6, Philadelphia, PA 19104, USA
* Corresponding author.
E-mail address: mitchele@chop.edu

Gastroenterol Clin N Am 52 (2023) 609–627
https://doi.org/10.1016/j.gtc.2023.05.009
0889-8553/23/© 2023 Elsevier Inc. All rights reserved.

health maintenance in patients with pIBD is essential. Studies have shown that patients with IBD are less likely to receive preventative care than otherwise healthy patients and even when received, there is a great variation.[12–17] In pediatrics, this is particularly complex because there are limited data to support recommendations and practice is often extrapolated from adult care.[9,11,12]

A multidisciplinary approach with a strong partnership between the gastroenterologist (GI) and primary care provider (PCP) is necessary to ensure appropriate health maintenance is received. Adult GI societies have published guidelines for health maintenance practices.[10,18] Recently, the Crohn's and Colitis Foundation's National Scientific Advisory Committee created publicly available, evidence-based health maintenance checklists for both adult and pediatric patients with IBD with resources that can guide the GI provider.[19]

Here, we review the important field of health-care maintenance in pIBD, exploring the risks, complications, and comorbidities as well as the literature to support current health maintenance practices.

ROUTINE VISITS AND DISEASE SURVEILLANCE

Essential to the health maintenance of patients with pIBD is routine visits with their GI provider along with a multidisciplinary team that may include a dietician, psychologist, and social worker.

Outpatient Clinic Visits

There are no established guidelines for how often a patient with pIBD should be seen by their GI provider. The frequency of visits is related to time from IBD diagnosis, disease activity, and dependent on maintenance therapy. Patients should continue to have regular visits with their GI provider even at times of disease quiescence but, importantly, these visits should not take the place of their regular PCP visits.

Disease Surveillance

Indirect measurements of disease activity can be achieved with monitoring of laboratories and fecal calprotectin (**Table 1**). Additional nutritional screening should also be periodically assessed (**Table 2**). In patients in remission on biologic or small-molecule

Table 1
Indirect markers for disease surveillance

Basic Laboratories	Evidence of Active IBD
CBC	Elevated white blood cell count Anemia (microcytic or normocytic) Elevated platelet count
Basic metabolic panel	Elevated blood urea nitrogen (BUN) to creatinine ratio Acidosis

Liver function panel	Hypoalbuminemia
	Elevated aspartate aminotransferase (AST),
	  alanine aminotransferase (ALT),
	  gamma-glutamyl transferase (GGT)

Inflammatory markers	Elevated C-reactive protein Elevated sedimentation rate
Stool studies	
Stool calprotectin	Elevated

Table 2
Nutritional deficiencies to consider in patients with pediatric inflammatory bowel disease

	Risk Factors	Symptoms	Diagnosis
Vitamin B12	Active ileitis, ileal resection, ileal pouch anal anastomosis	Megaloblastic anemia, pancytopenia, peripheral neuropathy, dementia	B12 < 200 pg/mL Elevated methylmalonic acid Elevated homocysteine level
Folate (B9)	Inadequate intake, malabsorption, ileitis, small bowel resection, medications (ie, methotrexate)	Megaloblastic anemia, glossitis, angular stomatitis, depression	Folate <2.5 ng/mL Elevated homocysteine level
Iron	Inadequate dietary intake, chronic blood loss, impaired iron absorption	Microcytic anemia, decreased exercise tolerance, tachycardia, pallor, angular cheilitis, glossitis, nausea, restless leg syndrome, depression	Transferrin saturation <20% Serum ferritin <30 (inactive disease) Serum ferritin <100 (active disease)
Vitamin D	Inadequate dietary intake, decreased sun exposure, fat malabsorption, bile salt deficiency (use of cholestyramine)	Decreased bone density, may increase disease activity/inflammation	Vitamin D 25 OH <15 = deficiency <30 = insufficiency ≥30 = sufficient/goal
Calcium	Inadequate dietary intake, vitamin D deficiency	Decreased bone density, muscle cramps, hypertension, hypoparathyroidism	DEXA scan, calcium level may not be reflective
Zinc	Chronic diarrhea, malabsorption	Acrodermatitis, poor wound healing	No accurate measurement, use clinical assessment

therapy, we recommend laboratories every 3 to 4 months. In patients close to diagnosis, starting a new therapy, and/or with active disease, laboratories may be drawn more often. For patients with mild disease and not on immunosuppressive therapy, laboratories can be drawn less frequently.

Fecal calprotectin is a useful indirect measure of bowel inflammation that can help monitor for active disease after diagnosis and to assess response to therapy. The trend can be very helpful but it does not take the place of endoscopic assessment.[20,21] It is important to note that elevations in fecal calprotectin are not always specific to IBD and can occur with infection, intestinal blood, inflammatory polyp, NSAID use, or malignancy.[21]

Direct assessment of disease is through endoscopy and augmented by radiologic evaluation. Pediatric groups recommend total colonoscopy with ileal intubation, upper endoscopy, multiple biopsies, and small bowel evaluation with imaging at diagnosis.[22,23] Endoscopic and mucosal healing is the goal of therapy and has been shown to decrease risk for hospitalization, surgery, disease complications, and growth failure.[24–26] There is growing consensus that repeat endoscopy should be performed after initiation of therapy to assess for mucosal healing, although there is not consensus regarding ideal timeframe, and benefit of early mucosal assessment must be weighed against the challenges of colonoscopy in pediatric patients. If disease is active or therapy must be changed, endoscopic evaluation is essential.

IMMUNIZATIONS

Receipt of proper immunizations is a cornerstone to health maintenance and prevention in all children and adolescents. In pediatric patients with IBD, it is especially important given baseline immune dysregulation and receipt of immunosuppressing therapies.[9,11] Despite the well-known risk of infection in patients with pIBD, rates of vaccination are insufficient.[27–29] **Table 3** outlines the vaccines to be received with additional pIBD considerations.

Special Considerations in Pediatric Inflammatory Bowel Disease

Live vaccinations should be avoided in immunosuppressed patients with pIBD based on criteria outlined in **Box 1**.[30–32] Efforts should be made to vaccinate young patients with live vaccinations before starting immunosuppressive therapy. Vaccination with live vaccines should occur at least 4 to 6 weeks before starting immunosuppressive therapy. If a patient is already on immunosuppression, live vaccines should not be given until 3 months after discontinuation of therapy.[30–32]

In some patients with pIBD, there are additional vaccinations that should be given. Patients with IBD, especially those on steroids, immunomodulators, or biologic or small-molecule therapies are at increased risk for the development of pneumococcal pneumonia.[33] Patients should receive additional pneumococcal vaccine based on Centers for Disease Control and Prevention (CDC) guidelines (see **Table 3**).[9]

Studies have shown that patients with IBD are also at an increased risk for developing herpes zoster (shingles).[34–36] Although the highest risk is in older patients, it is also increased in younger patients.[37] Risk of shingles is independently associated with immunosuppressive medications including steroids, anti-TNF therapy, and thiopurines.[35,37] More recently, tofacitinib has been shown to have increased risk of shingles, and the magnitude of risk is higher than with other immunosuppressive therapies.[10,36] Administration of the recombinant adjuvanted zoster vaccine, Shingrix, should be considered in patients aged 18 years or greater receiving Janus kinase (JAK) inhibitors, such as tofacitinib. In patients

Table 3
Vaccinations and important considerations in patients with pediatric inflammatory bowel disease

Vaccine Type	Live/Inactivated	Patient Population	Dosing Regimen	Special Considerations
Hepatitis A	Inactivated	All patients with IBD receive	2 doses at 0 and 6 mo	—
Hepatitis B (HBV)	Inactivated	All patients with IBD receive	3 doses at 0, 1, and 6 mo	• Before starting biologic therapy, check titers (anti-Hepatitis B surface antigen (HBsAg), anti-HBc (Hepatitis B core), HBsAg) • If not immune, repeat series • Recheck anti-HBsAg in patients requiring repeat series (1–2 mo after last dose) • If no response to revaccination, administer double Hepatitis B vaccine (HBV vaccine) or combination hepatitis A/B
Diphtheria, tetanus, pertussis (DTaP)	Inactivated	All patients with IBD receive	5 doses at 2, 4, 6, and 15–18 mo then 4–6 y old	• DTaP given if < 7 y old • Tdap can be administered at age 11–64 y with Td booster every 10 y
Meningococcal	Inactivated	All patients with IBD receive	2 doses at 11–2 y and 16 y old	—
Hemophilus influenzae type B	Inactivated	All patients with IBD receive	4 doses at 2, 4, 6, and 12–15 mo	—

(continued on next page)

Table 3
(continued)

Vaccine Type	Live/Inactivated	Patient Population	Dosing Regimen	Special Considerations
Poliovirus	Inactivated	All patients with IBD receive	4 doses at 2, 4, 6–18 mo and 4–6 y old	—
Human Papilloma virus	Inactivated	All patients with IBD aged 11–26 y old	3 doses at 0, 1, and 6 mo	—
Pneumococcal (PCV13 = Prevnar, PPSV23 = Preumovax)	Inactivated	Special consideration for patients with IBD	4 doses of PCV13 at 2, 4, 6, and 12–15 mo	• In immunocompromised patients ≥2 y old who have received PCV13 series: give PPSV23 at least 8 wk after any earlier pneumococcal vaccine dose • In immunocompromised patients 2–5 y old who have *not* received PCV13: 2 doses of PCV13 separated by 8 wk then PPSV23 at least 8 wk after second dose of PCV13 • In immunocompromised patients ≥6–18 y old who have *not* received PCV13: single dose of PCV13 then PPSV23 at least 8 wk later *Should receive PCV13 before giving any recommended doses of PPSV23* *Second PPSV23 dose given 5 y after the first PPSV23 Pediatric patients should not receive more than 2 doses of PPSV23 before 65 y of age*

Measles, Mumps, Rubella	Live	Contraindicated in immunosuppressed patients with IBD	2 doses at 12–15 mo and 4–6 y old	• Administer 2 doses 4 wk apart at least 6 wk before starting immunosuppressive therapy
Varicella	Live	Contraindicated in immunosuppressed patients with IBD	2 doses at 12–15 mo and 4–6 y old	• Before starting biologic therapy, assess for evidence of immunity: 1. Documentation of 2 doses; 2. Verification of diagnosis of varicella/herpes zoster by provider; 3. Varicella IgG antibody titer
Rotavirus	Live	Contraindicated in immunosuppressed patients with IBD	3 doses at 2, 4, and 6 mo	—
Herpes Zoster (Shingrix)	Inactivated	Special consideration for patients with IBD aged ≥18 y		• Consider in patients on JAK inhibitors or other high levels of immunosuppression
Influenza	Inactivated (intramuscular) Live (intranasal)	All patients with IBD to receive ≥6 mo old Contraindicated in immunosuppressed patients with IBD	Annual —	• Household members should be vaccinated
COVID-19	Inactivated (mRNA type)	Most patients with IBD eligible if ≥ 6 mo old	Initial series: 2 doses (3–4 wk between doses based on vaccine type)	• In immunocompromised: third dose 4 wk after second to complete initial series • Additional booster shots in children ≥5 y old per CDC recommendations

> **Box 1**
> **Criteria for immunosuppression in patients with special vaccine considerations**
>
> 1. Treatment with steroids of more than 20 mg/d (or equivalent of 2 mg/kg if <10 kg) EBM for 2 weeks *or* within 3 mo of stopping steroid therapy
>
> 2. Treatment with thiopurine, methotrexate, antitumor necrosis factor alpha agents or other biologic/small molecule *or* within 3 months of stopping these therapies
>
> 3. Significant protein-calorie malnutrition

receiving a combination of immunosuppression, this vaccine should also be considered on an individual basis.[10]

Influenza

Studies have shown that patients with IBD who are immunosuppressed are at an increased risk for influenza as compared with age-matched controls without IBD.[16,38] In addition, patients can experience a more severe course leading to hospitalization and superimposed bacterial pneumonia.[38,39] It is therefore important that patients with pIBD and household members are vaccinated against influenza annually. Studies in pediatrics and adults have shown adequate response to influenza vaccine, regardless of IBD medication regimen and timing relative to receipt of IBD therapy.[40–42]

Novel Coronavirus-19

Vaccination against the novel coronavirus-19 (COVID-19) provides the best protection against COVID-19. Although patients with IBD were not included in COVID-19 vaccination trials, in early 2021, the International Organization for the Study of Inflammatory Bowel Disease recommended that all eligible patients with IBD receive the COVID-19 vaccine.[43]

There have been concerns that initial rates of seroconversion and sustained antibody protection may be affected by immunosuppression in patients with IBD. Large multicenter trials in adults have shown variation in antibody level based on IBD therapy. In one prospective study, antibody concentrations were significantly lower in adult patients with IBD treated with infliximab (geometric mean ratio 0.21, 95% CI 0.08–0.17) and tofacitinib (0.43, 95% CI 0.23–0.81) as well as those of older age (0.79, 95% CI 0.72–0.87).[44] In another multicenter study, patients on anti-TNF therapy (OR 4.2, 95% CI 2.4–7.3) and those of older age (2.1, 95% CI 1.0–3.0) were more likely to have a blunted response to vaccination.[45] Despite these findings, overall studies in patients with IBD suggest low rates of breakthrough COVID-19 infection and relatively mild course of illness after vaccination.[46]

CDC recommendations for COVID-19 vaccination in children and adolescents are included in **Table 3**. The CDC currently recommends that patients considered moderately to severely immunocompromised receive an additional dose to complete the primary series as well as booster shots. In a recent study, patients with IBD who received an additional vaccine dose showed improved immunogenicity, even in those who had undetectable antibody levels after their initial series, with minimal side effects.[47]

GROWTH AND BONE HEALTH
Growth Failure

Growth failure is a unique aspect of pIBD and can influence treatment decisions and quality of life.[26] Malabsorption of nutrients, chronic inflammation, and steroid exposure contribute to growth failure. Growth failure can involve delays in both skeletal maturity and puberty.[48] Optimization of growth in children with pIBD is important because there is often a short window for intervention before the cessation of puberty and the pubertal growth spurt. Accurate assessment of height and weight at diagnosis and at subsequent follow-up visits, including a standardized z-score for age and sex, is important. If a patient is noted to have slowing of their growth, poor weight gain, and/or delay in pubertal development, further evaluation should be pursued to ensure that disease is not active.[11] Treatment with infliximab and surgical resection has been shown to significantly improve growth, mainly because of mucosal healing.[26,49] This is also likely true for other biologic agents as well, although data are limited. Involvement by a pediatric endocrinologist for growth failure may be appropriate in certain cases, especially when growth hormone is being considered.

Bone Health

Children and adolescents with IBD can have low bone density and altered bone structure, leading to a decrease in skeletal strength, increase in fracture risk, and compromise of linear growth.[50,51] Patients with IBD are at 40% increased risk of fracture as compared with age and sex-matched controls without IBD.[50] Nutritional deficiencies, decreased physical activity, increased inflammation, decreased muscle mass, and steroid exposure are factors that influence bone health in patients with IBD.[52–54] Deficits in bone mass can occur at the time of diagnosis but can also be acquired during the course of disease.[52]

Dual energy X-ray absorptiometry (DEXA) scan is the most well-accepted tool to measure bone mineral density.[11,51,52] Bone density is expressed as a z-score, which provides standardized values for age and sex.[52] It is well accepted that a DEXA scan should be performed at diagnosis to obtain baseline bone density measures.[52] However, the timing at which follow-up scans should be performed, if at all, is not well established. Follow-up scans should be based on initial DEXA results and disease course. A DEXA z-score of less than −2 represents significant deficits in bone mass and should prompt referral to a bone health expert as well as evaluation with bone age and laboratories. Subsequent DEXA scan should be performed, typically within 1 to 2 years, although timing is provider-dependent.[11,52] Patients with initial DEXA z-score less than −1 are considered to have borderline low bone mineral density and should be monitored with bone health evaluation based on risk factors, disease activity, and fracture history.[51,52] In patients with a normal DEXA scan at baseline, interval DEXA should be considered if certain risk factors develop including decrease in height or weight velocity, prolonged steroid exposure, amenorrhea, or significant fractures.[9,51,52]

There is no consensus on treatment of patients with pIBD with low bone density. Study with a bone health expert is essential. Optimization of dietary calcium and vitamin D with regular weight-bearing activities is first-line therapy. Bisphosphonates can be used in certain settings based on recommendations by a bone health expert.[9,11,51] Notably, anti-TNF therapy has been shown to improve bone density and thus bone health should be considered when deciding on therapy.[26,49,55] GI providers should counsel patients on ways to prevent bone disease (**Box 2**).[51]

NUTRITION

Nutritional support with a trained dietician and close monitoring of calorie and nutrient intake is important. Children with IBD are at an increased risk for macronutrient and micronutrient deficiencies, many of which are outlined in **Table 2**.[56] Although there

---

Box 2
Bone health maintenance and prevention practices

1. Ensure adequate consumption of calcium

2. Optimize vitamin D level with goal 30 to 50 ng/mL

3. Maintain normal body mass index (BMI) range

4. Increase in weight-bearing activities

5. Avoidance of medications that are known to negatively influence bone health

6. Periodic assessment for comorbidities that can negatively influence bone health

---

are no established guidelines for screening in pIBD, consideration of individual risk factors based on symptoms, distribution of disease, previous surgical history, and therapy can help to guide screening.[57–60]

Anemia and Iron Deficiency

Anemia is one of the most common yet underrecognized complications of IBD. The incidence in pIBD is 78%, higher than in adults with IBD.[61,62] There are often multiple contributing factors including iron deficiency anemia, anemia of chronic disease, vitamin deficiencies, hemolysis, and medication side effects.[63] Anemia and iron deficiency have been associated with increased rates of hospitalization and surgery as well as decreased quality of life, independent of disease activity.[64–67]

The North American Society for Pediatric GI, Hepatology and Nutrition recently published recommendations for anemia and iron deficiency screening. Patients with active disease should be screened every 3 months and those with inactive disease, every 6 to 12 months. Vitamin B12 and folate monitoring should occur annually.[63] Testing should include complete blood count (CBC), iron, total iron binding capacity, and ferritin. In an effort to improve screening and treatment rates, our IBD Center created an available clinical pathway (https://www.chop.edu/clinical-pathway/iron-deficiency-anemia-inflammatory-bowel-disease-ibd-clinical-pathway) with an integrated electronic medical record dashboard. We showed improvement in rates of iron deficiency screening and treatment as well as decreased prevalence of anemia.[64]

Treatment of anemia and iron deficiency should be based on the severity, availability of medications, medication side effects, and patient tolerance. In patients with mild and/or inactive disease, oral iron can be trialed initially. Parenteral iron can be used if a patient has severe iron deficiency, active disease, minimal response to oral iron, or intolerance to oral iron. Optimization of IBD therapy should also be considered.[63]

EYE DISEASE

Patients can have eye involvement as an extraintestinal manifestation of their IBD. The prevalence in pIBD is lower than in adults and is estimated between 0.6% and 1.8%.[68–71] The most common eye disease in pIBD is uveitis.[68] Children with Crohn Disease (CD) have 2.7 greater odds of eye disease as compared with children with ulcerative colitis (UC) and IBD-unclassified.[68] Some ophthalmologic manifestations can be related to disease activity, such as episcleritis, and others are independent, such as uveitis. In addition, there can be treatment-related ophthalmologic consequences.[68,70,71] Although ocular complications are rare, prevalence is thought to be underestimated as many patients can be asymptomatic. Studies evaluating routine ophthalmologic assessment have identified mild asymptomatic uveitis in 1.1% to 23% of patients.[68,72–74] In one pediatric study, 1.1% of patients had uveitis on routine examination and 7.4% had other abnormal ocular findings, although not all were thought to be primarily related to IBD.[74]

Surveillance is recommended, and although there is no consensus on frequency of surveillance, every 1 to 2 years has been suggested.[9,19] An ophthalmologic examination should include visual acuity, slit lamp examination, measurement of intraocular pressure, and examination of both the anterior and posterior chambers.[9] GI providers should educate patients and their caregivers on the increased risk of ocular involvement and the signs and symptoms.

SKIN HEALTH

There are multiple skin-related manifestations of IBD and consequences of immunosuppressive therapy that can occur. In this section, we will focus on skin cancer prevention and surveillance.

There is minimal data in pediatrics because skin cancer is extremely rare in this population. Data from adults have shown that patients with IBD are at an increased risk for the development of both melanoma and nonmelanoma skin cancer (NMSC), mainly basal and squamous cell carcinoma.[75,76] In one large retrospective cohort and nested case-control study, the incidence rate ratio (IRR) for melanoma and NMSC were increased in patients with IBD, 1.29 (95% CI 1.09–1.53) and 1.46 (1.40–1.53), respectively.[76] Suggested risk factors for the development of melanoma include anti-TNF exposure, CD, as well as extent and severity of disease.[76,77] Risk factors for NMSC include thiopurine exposure and anti-TNF therapy, with combination therapy yielding the highest risk.[76,78]

In pIBD, skin health maintenance capitalizes on prevention with focus on sun protection and avoidance. Patients should be counseled to seek shade, limit outdoor activities at peak sun times, wear sun-protective clothing, and use sunscreen.[9,19] Dermatologic evaluations are recommended, particularly in patients on immunosuppression, suspicious lesions or history of skin cancer.[19]

COLORECTAL CANCER SCREENING AND PREVENTION

The increased risk of colorectal cancer (CRC) is well accepted in patients with IBD. Risk for CRC increases in patients with longer duration of disease, increased degree of inflammation and extent of colitis, coexistent primary sclerosing cholangitis (PSC), and family history of CRC.[79,80] Although rare in pediatric patients, a large cohort study in Sweden reported an 18-fold increased risk of CRC in pIBD.[81] One recent retrospective pediatric study evaluated the incidence and characteristics of patients with pIBD who were subsequently diagnosed with CRC. Four of 443 were diagnosed with CRC, an incidence of 1.29 per 1000 person years, with median time from IBD to CRC diagnosis of 9.4 years. The sigmoid colon was most often involved, and adenocarcinoma was the most common histologic type.[82]

Cancer screening via colonoscopy should begin 8 to 10 years from the time of symptom-onset and should be performed every 1 to 3 years in patients with ulcerative colitis (UC) and Crohn Disease (CD) with at least one-third of their colon involved.[9,19,83] In patients with both UC and PSC, annual to biannual colonoscopy with biopsies for colon cancer surveillance should be performed.[9,19]

MENTAL HEALTH

Patients with pIBD are at an increased risk for depression, anxiety, adjustment disorder, altered self-image, school absences, family conflict, and issues with medication compliance.[84] In one study, patients with pIBD had higher rates of depression compared with controls, even compared with children with other chronic disease.[85] IBD presents unique challenges that affect self-esteem and social function. Increased disease severity has been shown to have a negative influence on quality of life and parental stress as well as an association with depression and anxiety.[84,86] In addition, depression can lead to greater pain and parent pain catastrophizing.[87]

It is important that GI providers are aware of these psychosocial issues. Increased fatigue, decreased energy, and decreased appetite could be due to active IBD but mood disorder should also be considered as a cause. It is recommended that a routine assessment to screen for depression and anxiety be performed at least annually in teenagers and young adults. These screens should be done more routinely when symptoms are present.[9,19] Access to a multidisciplinary team, including psychology and social work is important.[84]

SUBSTANCE USE

Rates of substance use are similar in patients with pIBD as compared with their same-aged peers.[88–90] In one survey-based study, 13% of adolescents with pIBD reported tobacco use, 23% marijuana use, and 34% binge drinking in the past 30 days.[88] Substance use has been associated with more active disease, increased hospitalization, decreased quality of life, poor psychosocial outcomes, and difficulty with medication adherence.[12,88] Motivation for substance use is often to treat IBD-related symptoms.[91] Despite this high prevalence of substance use in the pIBD population and associations with negative outcomes, 40% of adolescents with IBD report that their GI provider and PCP have not discussed substance use with them.[12] It is important that GIs provide anticipatory guidance and discuss the risks of substance use with their patients when appropriate.

HORMONAL CONTRACEPTION

IBD is often diagnosed during the reproductive years. Evidence-based reproductive counseling is important for young woman, although in one study, only 50% of adolescents reported that fertility and hormonal contraception (HC) were addressed by their GI or primary care providers.[12,92] It is important to discuss HC with adolescent patients with pIBD based on safety, IBD-related factors, and the patient's lifestyle.[93,94] A major consideration is that active IBD as well as use of estrogen-containing HC are associated with an increased risk for venous thromboembolism; as such, alternative forms of HC are important to consider.[95] HC can positively influence health and well-being and has been shown to improve menstrual-related IBD symptoms.[94,96]

Most medications used in pIBD do not affect fertility or fetal safety, although data are limited.[94] However, in patients requiring methotrexate, counseling about risk of associated teratogenicity should be provided and HC should be advised in sexually active young women.[94]

TRANSITION

Finally, critical to routine health maintenance in patients with pIBD is a smooth transition from pediatric to adult GI care. Patients with a more positive transition to an adult provider are more likely to engage in collaborative medical decision-making and have overall long-term management success.[97,98] Despite the clear benefits to a well-organized transition, most providers do not report the tools necessary to facilitate transition and most patients do not demonstrate transition readiness skills.[97] It is recommended that discussion about transition is approached early on, patients have the necessary tools to make the transition, and multispecialty involvement, including social work, occurs.[99]

SUMMARY

Patients with pIBD are at risk for multiple complications and comorbidities related to their immune dysregulation and immunosuppressive therapies. These issues include infection, nutritional deficiencies, growth and/or pubertal delay and failure, bone health, eye disease, and malignancy. IBD can also affect psychosocial well-being, substance use, and reproductive health.[9,11] A cornerstone to caring for patients with pIBD is to provide preventative care. Studies have shown that patients with pIBD are less likely to seek out and receive preventative care as compared with healthy patients.[12–17] Therefore, GI providers should work alongside PCPs to ensure that patients with pIBD are receiving health-care maintenance and monitoring. In addition, a multidisciplinary team is essential. Although practice is variable and data are limited in pIBD, this section summarizes the data that supports our health maintenance practice. Further emphasis on health maintenance and improving preventative care in pIBD is necessary.

CLINICS CARE POINTS

- Patients with pIBD are at increased risk for developing complications and comorbidities-Studies have shown that patients with IBD are less likely to receive preventative care and even when received, there is great variation in this care.
- Patients should be seen regularly by their GI provider with routine labs, imaging, and endoscopic evaluation based on timing from diagnosis, disease activity, and the type of maintenance therapy being received.
- Receipt of proper immunizations is important in pIBD and there are specific considerations that should be followed based on the age of the patient and the therapy being received-Patients with pIBD can have growth failure and poor bone health. Use of DEXA scan, at least at baseline, and optimization of bone health is essential.
- Children and adolescents with IBD are at increased risk for macronutrient and micronutrient deficiencies. It is important to screen for these deficiencies. Anemia and iron deficiency are of the most common yet underrecognized complications of pIBD.Recognition and treatment for this is important.
- There are multiple eye and skin related manifestation of pIBD and surveillance is recommended
- There is increased risk of colorectal cancer in patients with IBD. Cancer screening via colonoscopy should begin 8-10 years from the time of symptom-onset and should be performed every 1-3 years in patients with UC and/or CD with at least 1/3 of their colon involved. Annual to biannual colonoscopy with biopsies should be performed in patients with UC and PSC
- Screening for issues related to mental health and substance use should be instituted into pIBD practice. Evidence-based reproductive health counseling is also important
- Transition from pediatric to adult GI care is important and should be approached early on, providing patients with the necessary tools to make the transition with multispecialty involvement
- GI providers should work alongside PCPs to ensure that patients with pIBD are receiving health-care maintenance and monitoring. A multidisciplinary team is essential and further emphasize and improvement in this area is needed.

DISCLOSURE

The authors have nothing to disclose.

REFERENCES

1. Sartor RB. Mechanisms of disease: pathogenesis of Crohn's disease and ulcerative colitis. Nat Clin Pract Gastroenterol Hepatol 2006;3:390–407.
2. Ye Y, Manne S, Treem WR, et al. Prevalence of Inflammatory Bowel Disease in Pediatric and Adult Populations: Recent Estimates From Large National Databases in the United States, 2007-2016. Inflamm Bowel Dis 2020;26:619–25.
3. Benchimol EI, Bernstein CN, Bitton A, et al. Trends in Epidemiology of Pediatric Inflammatory Bowel Disease in Canada: Distributed Network Analysis of Multiple Population-Based Provincial Health Administrative Databases. Am J Gastroenterol 2017;112:1120–34.
4. Malmborg P, Grahnquist L, Lindholm J, et al. Increasing incidence of paediatric inflammatory bowel disease in northern Stockholm County, 2002-2007. J Pediatr Gastroenterol Nutr 2013;57:29–34.
5. Pigneur B, Seksik P, Viola S, et al. Natural history of Crohn's disease: comparison between childhood- and adult-onset disease. Inflamm Bowel Dis 2010;16:953–61.
6. Rosen MJ, Dhawan A, Saeed SA. Inflammatory Bowel Disease in Children and Adolescents. JAMA Pediatr 2015;169:1053–60.
7. Turner D, Griffiths AM, Wilson D, et al. Designing clinical trials in paediatric inflammatory bowel diseases: a PIBDnet commentary. Gut 2020;69:32–41.
8. Van Limbergen J, Russell RK, Drummond HE, et al. Definition of phenotypic characteristics of childhood-onset inflammatory bowel disease. Gastroenterology 2008;135:1114–22.
9. DeFilippis EM, Sockolow R, Barfield E. Health Care Maintenance for the Pediatric Patient With Inflammatory Bowel Disease. Pediatrics 2016;138.
10. Syal G, Serrano M, Jain A, et al. Health Maintenance Consensus for Adults With Inflammatory Bowel Disease. Inflamm Bowel Dis 2021;27:1552–63.
11. Breglio KJ, Rosh JR. Health maintenance and vaccination strategies in pediatric inflammatory bowel disease. Inflamm Bowel Dis 2013;19:1740–4.
12. Michel HK, Kim SC, Siripong N, et al. Gaps Exist in the Comprehensive Care of Children with Inflammatory Bowel Diseases. J Pediatr 2020;224:94–101.
13. Michel HK, Noll RB, Siripong N, et al. Patterns of Primary, Specialty, Urgent Care, and Emergency Department Care in Children With Inflammatory Bowel Diseases. J Pediatr Gastroenterol Nutr 2020;71:e28–34.
14. Selby L, Hoellein A, Wilson JF. Are primary care providers uncomfortable providing routine preventive care for inflammatory bowel disease patients? Dig Dis Sci 2011;56:819–24.
15. Wasan SK, Coukos JA, Farraye FA. Vaccinating the inflammatory bowel disease patient: deficiencies in gastroenterologists knowledge. Inflamm Bowel Dis 2011;17:2536–40.
16. Mir FA, Kane SV. Health Maintenance in Inflammatory Bowel Disease. Curr Gastroenterol Rep 2018;20:23.
17. Selby L, Kane S, Wilson J, et al. Receipt of preventive health services by IBD patients is significantly lower than by primary care patients. Inflamm Bowel Dis 2008;14:253–8.
18. Farraye FA, Melmed GY, Lichtenstein GR, et al. ACG Clinical Guideline: Preventive Care in Inflammatory Bowel Disease. Am J Gastroenterol 2017;112:241–58.

19. Ghersin I, Khateeb N, Katz LH, et al. Anthropometric Measures in Adolescents With Inflammatory Bowel Disease: A Population-Based Study. Inflamm Bowel Dis 2019;25:1061–5.

20. Alibrahim B, Aljasser MI, Salh B. Fecal calprotectin use in inflammatory bowel disease and beyond: A mini-review. Can J Gastroenterol Hepatol 2015;29:157–63.

21. Vernia F, Di Ruscio M, Stefanelli G, et al. Is fecal calprotectin an accurate marker in the management of Crohn's disease? J Gastroenterol Hepatol 2020;35: 390–400.

22. Ibd Working Group of the European Society for Paediatric Gastroenterology H, Nutrition. Inflammatory bowel disease in children and adolescents: recommendations for diagnosis–the Porto criteria. J Pediatr Gastroenterol Nutr 2005;41:1–7.

23. Levine A, Turner D, Pfeffer Gik T, et al. Comparison of outcomes parameters for induction of remission in new onset pediatric Crohn's disease: evaluation of the porto IBD group "growth relapse and outcomes with therapy" (GROWTH CD) study. Inflamm Bowel Dis 2014;20:278–85.

24. Bouguen G, Levesque BG, Feagan BG, et al. Treat to target: a proposed new paradigm for the management of Crohn's disease. Clin Gastroenterol Hepatol 2015;13:1042–10450.e2.

25. Shah SC, Colombel JF, Sands BE, et al. Systematic review with meta-analysis: mucosal healing is associated with improved long-term outcomes in Crohn's disease. Aliment Pharmacol Ther 2016;43:317–33.

26. Walters TD, Kim MO, Denson LA, et al. Increased effectiveness of early therapy with anti-tumor necrosis factor-alpha vs an immunomodulator in children with Crohn's disease. Gastroenterology 2014;146:383–91.

27. Longuet R, Willot S, Ginies JL, et al. Immunization status in children with inflammatory bowel disease. Eur J Pediatr 2014;173:603–8.

28. Martinelli M, Giugliano FP, Strisciuglio C, et al. Vaccinations and Immunization Status in Pediatric Inflammatory Bowel Disease: A Multicenter Study From the Pediatric IBD Porto Group of the ESPGHAN. Inflamm Bowel Dis 2020;26:1407–14.

29. Wasan SK, Calderwood AH, Long MD, et al. Immunization rates and vaccine beliefs among patients with inflammatory bowel disease: an opportunity for improvement. Inflamm Bowel Dis 2014;20:246–50.

30. Rahier JF, Magro F, Abreu C, et al. Second European evidence-based consensus on the prevention, diagnosis and management of opportunistic infections in inflammatory bowel disease. J Crohns Colitis 2014;8:443–68.

31. Sands BE, Cuffari C, Katz J, et al. Guidelines for immunizations in patients with inflammatory bowel disease. Inflamm Bowel Dis 2004;10:677–92.

32. Veereman-Wauters G, de Ridder L, Veres G, et al. Risk of infection and prevention in pediatric patients with IBD: ESPGHAN IBD Porto Group commentary. J Pediatr Gastroenterol Nutr 2012;54:830–7.

33. Long MD, Martin C, Sandler RS, et al. Increased risk of pneumonia among patients with inflammatory bowel disease. Am J Gastroenterol 2013;108:240–8.

34. Khan N, Patel D, Trivedi C, et al. Overall and Comparative Risk of Herpes Zoster With Pharmacotherapy for Inflammatory Bowel Diseases: A Nationwide Cohort Study. Clin Gastroenterol Hepatol 2018;16:1919–19127.e3.

35. Long MD, Martin C, Sandler RS, et al. Increased risk of herpes zoster among 108 604 patients with inflammatory bowel disease. Aliment Pharmacol Ther 2013;37: 420–9.

36. Winthrop KL, Melmed GY, Vermeire S, et al. Herpes Zoster Infection in Patients With Ulcerative Colitis Receiving Tofacitinib. Inflamm Bowel Dis 2018;24:2258–65.

37. Gupta G, Lautenbach E, Lewis JD. Incidence and risk factors for herpes zoster among patients with inflammatory bowel disease. Clin Gastroenterol Hepatol 2006;4:1483–90.

38. Stobaugh DJ, Deepak P, Ehrenpreis ED. Hospitalizations for vaccine preventable pneumonias in patients with inflammatory bowel disease: a 6-year analysis of the Nationwide Inpatient Sample. Clin Exp Gastroenterol 2013;6:43–9.

39. Tinsley A, Navabi S, Williams ED, et al. Increased Risk of Influenza and Influenza-Related Complications Among 140,480 Patients With Inflammatory Bowel Disease. Inflamm Bowel Dis 2019;25:369–76.

40. Mamula P, Markowitz JE, Piccoli DA, et al. Immune response to influenza vaccine in pediatric patients with inflammatory bowel disease. Clin Gastroenterol Hepatol 2007;5:851–6.

41. Muller KE, Dohos D, Sipos Z, et al. Immune response to influenza and pneumococcal vaccines in adults with inflammatory bowel disease: A systematic review and meta-analysis of 1429 patients. Vaccine 2022;40:2076–86.

42. deBruyn J, Fonseca K, Ghosh S, et al. Immunogenicity of Influenza Vaccine for Patients with Inflammatory Bowel Disease on Maintenance Infliximab Therapy: A Randomized Trial. Inflamm Bowel Dis 2016;22:638–47.

43. Siegel CA, Melmed GY, McGovern DP, et al. SARS-CoV-2 vaccination for patients with inflammatory bowel diseases: recommendations from an international consensus meeting. Gut 2021;70:635–40.

44. Alexander JL, Kennedy NA, Ibraheim H, et al. COVID-19 vaccine-induced antibody responses in immunosuppressed patients with inflammatory bowel disease (VIP): a multicentre, prospective, case-control study. Lancet Gastroenterol Hepatol 2022;7:342–52.

45. Kappelman MD, Weaver KN, Zhang X, et al. Factors Affecting Initial Humoral Immune Response to SARS-CoV-2 Vaccines Among Patients With Inflammatory Bowel Diseases. Am J Gastroenterol 2022;117:462–9.

46. Weaver KN, Zhang X, Dai X, et al. Low Rates of Breakthrough COVID-19 Infection After SARS-CoV-2 Vaccination in Patients With Inflammatory Bowel Disease. Inflamm Bowel Dis 2023;29(3):483–6.

47. Long MD, Weaver KN, Zhang X, et al. Strong Response to SARS-CoV-2 Vaccine Additional Doses Among Patients With Inflammatory Bowel Diseases. Clin Gastroenterol Hepatol 2022;20:1881–1883 e1.

48. Heuschkel R, Salvestrini C, Beattie RM, et al. Guidelines for the management of growth failure in childhood inflammatory bowel disease. Inflamm Bowel Dis 2008; 14:839–49.

49. Hyams J, Crandall W, Kugathasan S, et al. Induction and maintenance infliximab therapy for the treatment of moderate-to-severe Crohn's disease in children. Gastroenterology 2007;132:863–73 [quiz: 1165–6].

50. Bernstein CN, Benchimol EI, Bitton A, et al. The Impact of Inflammatory Bowel Disease in Canada 2018: Extra-intestinal Diseases in IBD. J Can Assoc Gastroenterol 2019;2:S73–80.

51. Gordon RJ, Gordon CM. Bone Health in Pediatric Patients with IBD: What Is New? Curr Osteoporos Rep 2021;19:429–35.

52. Pappa H, Thayu M, Sylvester F, et al. Skeletal health of children and adolescents with inflammatory bowel disease. J Pediatr Gastroenterol Nutr 2011;53:11–25.

53. Ricciuto A, Aardoom M, Orlanski-Meyer E, et al. Predicting Outcomes in Pediatric Crohn's Disease for Management Optimization: Systematic Review and Consensus Statements From the Pediatric Inflammatory Bowel Disease-Ahead Program. Gastroenterology 2021;160:403–36.e26.

54. Ricciuto A, Mack DR, Huynh HQ, et al. Diagnostic Delay Is Associated With Complicated Disease and Growth Impairment in Paediatric Crohn's Disease. J Crohns Colitis 2021;15:419–31.
55. Thayu M, Leonard MB, Hyams JS, et al. Improvement in biomarkers of bone formation during infliximab therapy in pediatric Crohn's disease: results of the REACH study. Clin Gastroenterol Hepatol 2008;6:1378–84.
56. Hartman C, Eliakim R, Shamir R. Nutritional status and nutritional therapy in inflammatory bowel diseases. World J Gastroenterol 2009;15:2570–8.
57. Fritz J, Walia C, Elkadri A, et al. A Systematic Review of Micronutrient Deficiencies in Pediatric Inflammatory Bowel Disease. Inflamm Bowel Dis 2019;25:445–59.
58. Hwang C, Ross V, Mahadevan U. Micronutrient deficiencies in inflammatory bowel disease: from A to zinc. Inflamm Bowel Dis 2012;18:1961–81.
59. Pappa HM, Gordon CM, Saslowsky TM, et al. Vitamin D status in children and young adults with inflammatory bowel disease. Pediatrics 2006;118:1950–61.
60. Wu Z, Liu D, Deng F. The Role of Vitamin D in Immune System and Inflammatory Bowel Disease. J Inflamm Res 2022;15:3167–85.
61. Pels LP, Van de Vijver E, Waalkens HJ, et al. Slow hematological recovery in children with IBD-associated anemia in cases of "expectant management". J Pediatr Gastroenterol Nutr 2010;51:708–13.
62. Sjoberg D, Holmstrom T, Larsson M, et al. Anemia in a population-based IBD cohort (ICURE): still high prevalence after 1 year, especially among pediatric patients. Inflamm Bowel Dis 2014;20:2266–70.
63. Goyal A, Zheng Y, Albenberg LG, et al. Anemia in Children With Inflammatory Bowel Disease: A Position Paper by the IBD Committee of the North American Society of Pediatric Gastroenterology, Hepatology and Nutrition. J Pediatr Gastroenterol Nutr 2020;71:563–82.
64. Breton J, Witmer CM, Zhang Y, et al. Utilization of an Electronic Medical Record-integrated Dashboard Improves Identification and Treatment of Anemia and Iron Deficiency in Pediatric Inflammatory Bowel Disease. Inflamm Bowel Dis 2021;27:1409–17.
65. Danese S, Hoffman C, Vel S, et al. Anaemia from a patient perspective in inflammatory bowel disease: results from the European Federation of Crohn's and Ulcerative Colitis Association's online survey. Eur J Gastroenterol Hepatol 2014;26:1385–91.
66. Ershler WB, Chen K, Reyes EB, et al. Economic burden of patients with anemia in selected diseases. Value Health 2005;8:629–38.
67. Wells CW, Lewis S, Barton JR, et al. Effects of changes in hemoglobin level on quality of life and cognitive function in inflammatory bowel disease patients. Inflamm Bowel Dis 2006;12:123–30.
68. Ottaviano G, Salvatore S, Salvatoni A, et al. Ocular Manifestations of Paediatric Inflammatory Bowel Disease: A Systematic Review and Meta-analysis. J Crohns Colitis 2018;12:870–9.
69. Castro M, Papadatou B, Baldassare M, et al. Inflammatory bowel disease in children and adolescents in Italy: data from the pediatric national IBD register (1996-2003). Inflamm Bowel Dis 2008;14:1246–52.
70. Dotson JL, Hyams JS, Markowitz J, et al. Extraintestinal manifestations of pediatric inflammatory bowel disease and their relation to disease type and severity. J Pediatr Gastroenterol Nutr 2010;51:140–5.
71. Rohani P, Abdollah Gorji F, Eshaghi M, et al. Ocular Complications of Pediatric Inflammatory Bowel Disease: A Case Series From a Pediatric Tertiary Medical Center. Clin Pediatr (Phila) 2022;61:347–51.

72. Daum F, Gould HB, Gold D, et al. Asymptomatic transient uveitis in children with inflammatory bowel disease. Am J Dis Child 1979;133:170–1.

73. Hofley P, Roarty J, McGinnity G, et al. Asymptomatic uveitis in children with chronic inflammatory bowel diseases. J Pediatr Gastroenterol Nutr 1993;17: 397–400.

74. Naviglio S, Parentin F, Nider S, et al. Ocular Involvement in Children with Inflammatory Bowel Disease. Inflamm Bowel Dis 2017;23:986–90.

75. Long MD. Cutaneous malignancies in patients with inflammatory bowel disease. Gastroenterol Hepatol 2012;8:467–71.

76. Long MD, Martin CF, Pipkin CA, et al. Risk of melanoma and nonmelanoma skin cancer among patients with inflammatory bowel disease. Gastroenterology 2012; 143:390–399 e1.

77. Nissen LHC, Pierik M, Derikx L, et al. Risk Factors and Clinical Outcomes in Patients with IBD with Melanoma. Inflamm Bowel Dis 2017;23:2018–26.

78. Long MD, Herfarth HH, Pipkin CA, et al. Increased risk for non-melanoma skin cancer in patients with inflammatory bowel disease. Clin Gastroenterol Hepatol 2010;8:268–74.

79. Kim ER, Chang DK. Colorectal cancer in inflammatory bowel disease: the risk, pathogenesis, prevention and diagnosis. World J Gastroenterol 2014;20: 9872–81.

80. Wijnands AM, de Jong ME, Lutgens M, et al. Prognostic Factors for Advanced Colorectal Neoplasia in Inflammatory Bowel Disease: Systematic Review and Meta-analysis. Gastroenterology 2021;160:1584–98.

81. Olen O, Askling J, Sachs MC, et al. Childhood onset inflammatory bowel disease and risk of cancer: a Swedish nationwide cohort study 1964-2014. BMJ 2017; 358:j3951.

82. Kim MJ, Ko JS, Shin M, et al. Colorectal Cancer associated with pediatric inflammatory bowel disease: a case series. BMC Pediatr 2021;21:504.

83. Clarke WT, Feuerstein JD. Colorectal cancer surveillance in inflammatory bowel disease: Practice guidelines and recent developments. World J Gastroenterol 2019;25:4148–57.

84. Mackner LM, Greenley RN, Szigethy E, et al. Psychosocial issues in pediatric inflammatory bowel disease: report of the North American Society for Pediatric Gastroenterology, Hepatology, and Nutrition. J Pediatr Gastroenterol Nutr 2013; 56:449–58.

85. Keethy D, Mrakotsky C, Szigethy E. Pediatric inflammatory bowel disease and depression: treatment implications. Curr Opin Pediatr 2014;26:561–7.

86. Gray WN, Boyle SL, Graef DM, et al. Health-related quality of life in youth with Crohn disease: role of disease activity and parenting stress. J Pediatr Gastroenterol Nutr 2015;60:749–53.

87. Murphy LK, de la Vega R, Kohut SA, et al. Systematic Review: Psychosocial Correlates of Pain in Pediatric Inflammatory Bowel Disease. Inflamm Bowel Dis 2021; 27:697–710.

88. Plevinsky JM, Maddux MH, Greenley RN. Substance Use in Adolescents and Young Adults With Inflammatory Bowel Diseases: An Exploratory Cluster Analysis. J Pediatr Gastroenterol Nutr 2019;69:324–9.

89. Phatak UP, Rojas-Velasquez D, Porto A, et al. Prevalence and Patterns of Marijuana Use in Young Adults With Inflammatory Bowel Disease. J Pediatr Gastroenterol Nutr 2017;64:261–4.

90. Wisk LE, Weitzman ER. Substance Use Patterns Through Early Adulthood: Results for Youth With and Without Chronic Conditions. Am J Prev Med 2016;51: 33–45.
91. Hoffenberg EJ, Newman H, Collins C, et al. Cannabis and Pediatric Inflammatory Bowel Disease: Change Blossoms a Mile High. J Pediatr Gastroenterol Nutr 2017; 64:265–71.
92. Toomey D, Waldron B. Family planning and inflammatory bowel disease: the patient and the practitioner. Fam Pract 2013;30:64–8.
93. Gawron LM, Sanders J, Steele KP, et al. Reproductive Planning and Contraception for Women with Inflammatory Bowel Diseases. Inflamm Bowel Dis 2016;22: 459–64.
94. Martin J, Kane SV, Feagins LA. Fertility and Contraception in Women With Inflammatory Bowel Disease. Gastroenterol Hepatol 2016;12:101–9.
95. Peragallo Urrutia R, Coeytaux RR, McBroom AJ, et al. Risk of acute thromboembolic events with oral contraceptive use: a systematic review and meta-analysis. Obstet Gynecol 2013;122:380–9.
96. Gawron LM, Goldberger A, Gawron AJ, et al. The impact of hormonal contraception on disease-related cyclical symptoms in women with inflammatory bowel diseases. Inflamm Bowel Dis 2014;20:1729–33.
97. Gray WN, Maddux MH. Current Transition Practices in Pediatric IBD: Findings from a National Survey of Pediatric Providers. Inflamm Bowel Dis 2016;22:372–9.
98. Plevinsky JM, Gumidyala AP, Fishman LN. Transition experience of young adults with inflammatory bowel diseases (IBD): a mixed methods study. Child Care Health Dev 2015;41:755–61.
99. Steinberg JM, Charabaty A. The Management Approach to the Adolescent IBD Patient: Health Maintenance and Medication Considerations. Curr Gastroenterol Rep 2020;22:5.

Optimizing the Transition and Transfer of Care in Pediatric Inflammatory Bowel Disease

Laurie N. Fishman, MD[a,b,*], Julia Ding, MD[c]

KEYWORDS

- Inflammatory bowel disease • IBD • Transition care • Adolescent • Pediatrics
- Crohn disease • Ulcerative colitis

KEY POINTS

- Thoughtful transition of patients with inflammatory bowel disease (IBD) from pediatric to adult care is important in the success of transition and improves patient outcomes.
- Transition is a gradual process that can start at any age and culminates in the transfer to adult care.
- Optimizing care involves organizing age-appropriate development of self-management skills over time.
- Assessing readiness and transferring care can take on many forms; there is no uniform strategy but overall intentional planning will be beneficial.

INTRODUCTION

Transition care is a valuable field to help patients entering adult medical care to succeed with the knowledge and skills needed to navigate a new medical system and culture. Thoughtful consideration of the process can improve chances of a successful transition, and conversely lack of transition resources may lead to worse outcomes for patients.[1,2] Prioritizing health care transition (HCT) has been endorsed by the American Academy of Pediatrics, American Academy of Family Physicians, and the American College of Physicians.[3] Although the skills are valuable to all emerging young adults, they are especially so for those with a chronic illness such as

[a] Division of Gastroenterology and Nutrition, Boston Children's Hospital, 300 Longwood Avenue, Boston, MA 02115, USA; [b] Harvard Medical School, 25 Shattuck Street, Boston, MA 02115, USA; [c] Division of Gastroenterology and Hepatology, Boston University School of Medicine, 72 East Concord Street, Boston, MA 02118, USA
* Corresponding author.
E-mail address: Laurie.fishman@childrens.harvard.edu

Gastroenterol Clin N Am 52 (2023) 629–644
https://doi.org/10.1016/j.gtc.2023.05.004
0889-8553/23/© 2023 Elsevier Inc. All rights reserved.

inflammatory bowel disease (IBD), who need to navigate the health care system consistently with a complex disease.

HCT is best accomplished in a structured and consistent manner. The 6 core elements described by the widely used Got Transition program helps the practice or institution engage stakeholders and gives providers a roadmap for implementation (**Fig. 1**).[4]

The Got Transition approach and timeline for transition applies to all patients entering adulthood, even if they are maintaining rather than switching health care relationships such as is the case with medicine-pediatric and family medicine providers. Although transfer of care to adult providers may be cited as the rationale, the self-management skills developed in the transition process are universally beneficial. In this review the authors discuss the process of HCT and highlight concepts for optimizing the transition of care of patients with IBD moving from pediatric to adult medical care. Although a variety of different strategies and models have been proposed, lack of comparative outcome data has meant that there is no single definitive model.[5] However, there are numerous best practices that can be used from the growing literature on this topic.

IMPORTANCE OF TRANSITION CARE IN INFLAMMATORY BOWEL DISEASE

Approximately 25% of patients with IBD will be diagnosed before age 20 years, and the overall incidence of IBD is increasing around the world.[6,7] Patients with IBD who present in the pediatric age range tend to have more complex and severe disease.[8] These children will need ongoing care into adult years, ideally in a seamless fashion.

Planned transition has been shown to have significant effects on the medical course of the disease. Patients attending a transition program in Australia had less emergency department (ED) visits than those who had not gone through the program.[9] In an observational study encompassing 11 centers in the United Kingdom, patients who attended a structured transition program were more likely to be steroid-free or to avoid ED visits leading to admissions, in comparison with their historic controls.[10] Another study reported that patients who had undergone transition programs had better attendance for clinic visits, better medication adherence, optimal growth, and less surgery.[11] Recognition of the need for transition care is important because significant time and resources may be needed for HCT to be done in an optimal manner.

SETTING EXPECTATIONS

The goal of HCT is to have an organized coordinated process that will optimize health and prepare each patient for future sustainable success.[5] It is important to distinguish the process of transition from the later step of transfer to adult care. Transition is a gradual and intentional process by which the patient learns about their own disease,

SIX CORE ELEMENTS™ APPROACH AND TIMELINE FOR
YOUTH TRANSITIONING FROM PEDIATRIC TO ADULT HEALTH CARE

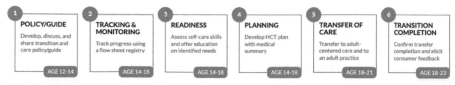

Fig. 1. Core elements of transition to adult health care.

takes responsibility for treatment, and communicates with providers during and between visits. Ideally, it would be a process that builds confidence for all stakeholders.

It can be helpful for patients and family to set the expectation early on that all patients will need to graduate from their pediatric provider. Age of transition may vary depending on personal and societal influences. In Europe and Canada, HCT typically occurs at age 18 years. In the United States, the age of transition varies more, typically occurring around age 18 to 21 years but without clear limits can be extended into adulthood.

When age is not the sole determinant of transfer, the clarity around timing disappears. There is discordance among health care providers about when the transition process should take place and what should be triggers or indications to require transfer.[12,13] Milestones, such as college graduation, marriage, steady employment, or starting a family, may be triggers for some providers to initiate transfer. Disruptive behavior, incarceration, or drug use may invoke anger or discomfort in the pediatric providers and unfortunately may result in a more abrupt transfer or earlier transfer. Unanticipated pregnancy might require precipitous transfer. Many pediatric providers quote "readiness" as the factor to use for transfer; however, the definition is not universal. The threshold for "readiness" has not been clarified even when this is used as a trigger. Ideally, the timing is defined in a way that can be anticipated and discussed for several years before the transfer, as would occur with age-based criteria. Using criteria other than age or milestones increases the possibility for unanticipated transfers. Anticipation and planning can improve the chances for a smooth and successful transfer of care.

DEVELOPING SELF-MANAGEMENT SKILLS

Transition, the slow movement toward self-management and autonomy, should be overtly discussed when patients are about 12 to 14 years old.[14] Transition task lists tend to group skills by age (**Fig. 2**), so providers can quickly assess developmentally appropriate topics and set expectations for behaviors. Screening strategies can be based on this information and incorporated into clinic flow or the electronic medical records. Integration of transition tools has been shown as an effective way to standardize and distribute self-assessments and skills practicums during patient visits, without significantly affecting clinical workflow. This system can carry forward progress between visits and be a reminder for topics to revisit at the following appointment.[14]

However, skills may also be conceptualized in content groupings, such as knowledge about condition, medication related skills, ability to communicate with providers during and outside of clinic, and navigation of the health care system. It may be easier for providers to sequence the teaching of tasks in this manner. Health care transition is most successful when there is a designated health care provider who is able to work collaboratively with the patient and family to take responsibility for the process.[5,15] With pediatric patients with IBD, it is often the pediatric gastroenterologist who plays a central role in initiation and pacing of transition, taking into account practical and emotional considerations.[16]

Patients with IBD should have knowledge about their own condition.[17,18] Scores for IBD knowledge vary depending on the number and type of questions asked; however, it is common to have adolescents achieve approximately 50% accuracy.[17,19,20] Studies have often found that male sex, lower educational level, less acceptance of disease, and increased dependence on parents correlate with lower disease knowledge.[17] Disease understanding will be needed to report medical history to providers and to

Healthcare Provider Transitioning Checklist

AGE	PATIENT	HEALTH CARE TEAM
12-14	**EARLY ADOLESCENCE** *New knowledge and responsibilities* ☐ I can describe my GI condition ☐ I can name my medications, the amount and times I take them ☐ I can describe the common side effects of my medications ☐ I know my doctors' and nurses' names and roles ☐ I can use and read a thermometer ☐ I can answer at least 1 question during my health care visit ☐ I can manage my regular medical tasks at school ☐ I can call my doctor's office to make or change an appointment ☐ I can describe how my GI condition affects me on a daily basis	☐ Discuss the idea of visiting the office without parents or guardians in the future ☐ Encourage independence by performing part of the exam with the parents or guardians out of the examining room ☐ Begin to provide information about drugs, alcohol, sexuality and fitness ☐ Establish specific self-management goals during office visit

14-17	**MID ADOLESCENCE**
	Building knowledge and practicing independence
	
	☐ I know the names and purposes of the tests that are done
	☐ I know what can trigger a flare of my disease
	☐ I know my medical history
	☐ I know if I need to transition to an adult gastroenterologist
	☐ I reorder my medications and call my doctor for refills
	☐ I answer many questions during a health care visit
	☐ I spend most of my time alone with the doctor during visit
	☐ I understand the risk of medical nonadherence
	☐ I understand the impact of drugs and alcohol on my condition
	☐ I understand the impact of my GI condition on my sexuality
		☐ Always focus on the patient instead of the parents or guardians when providing any explanations and
		☐ Allow the patient to select when the parent or guardian is in the room for the exam
		☐ Inform the patient of what the parent or guardian must legally be informed about with regards to the patient condition
		☐ Discuss the importance of preparing the patient for independent status with the parents or guardian and address any anxiety they may have
		☐ Continue to set specific goals which should include:
		  • Filling prescriptions and scheduling appointments
		  • Keeping a list of medications and medical team contact information in wallet and backpack

17+	**LATE ADOLESCENCE** *Taking charge* ☐ I can describe what medications I should not take because they might interact with the medications I am taking for my health condition ☐ I am alone with the doctor or choose who is with me during a health care visit ☐ I can tell someone what new legal rights and responsibilities I gained when I turned 18 ☐ I manage all my medical tasks outside the home (school, work) ☐ I know how to get more information about IBD ☐ I can book my own appointments, refill prescriptions and contact medical team ☐ I can tell someone how long I can be covered under my parents' health insurance plan and what I need to do to maintain coverage for the next 2 years ☐ I carry insurance information (card) with me in my wallet/purse/backpack	**DISCUSS IN MORE DEPTH:** ☐ The impact of drugs, alcohol and non adherence on their disease ☐ The impact of their disease on sexuality, fertility ☐ Future plans for school/work and impact on health care including insurance coverage ☐ How eventual transfer of care to an adult gastroenterologist will coordinate with future school or employment plans ☐ Remind patient and family that at age 18 the patient has the right to make his or her own health choices ☐ Develop specific plans for self-management outside the home (work/school) ☐ Provide the patient with a medical summary for work, school or transition ☐ Discuss plans for insurance coverage ☐ If transitioning to an adult subspecialist, provide a list of potential providers and encourage/facilitate an initial visit

Fig. 2. NASPGHAN transition checklist. (*From* NASPGHAN. NASPGHAN - Inflammatory Bowel Disease. Healthcare Provider Checklist for Transitioning a Patient from Pediatric to Adult Care. Available at https://naspghan.org/professional-resources/medical-professional-resources/inflammatory-bowel-disease/; with permission.)

self-monitor for complications. Increased disease knowledge has been linked to improved medication adherence.[18]

Medication management is an integral part to IBD care, as lapses in medication compliance may result in worse acute and long-term health outcomes. Adolescents with IBD generally have poor adherence to treatment, making this a particularly important area of focus.[18,21] Patients should be able to know the names and eventually the doses of their medicines and when to administer them. They should understand the timing of their standing and as-needed medications and be given graded autonomy in self-administering them. Picking up medications from the pharmacy and calling in refills can be a daunting challenge to an adolescent. Asking them to start with one part of the process, such as calling in a refill, can help boost confidence, especially if there is a family member nearby to provide support if needed. Skills to manage medications given as infusions and injections differ from oral medications and also need to be overtly taught to adolescents.[22]

Communication skills build gradually, with patients first learning to independently answer the physician questions during the visit. In one study, 55% of patients reported answering questions by age 16 years but at the same age only 15% asked questions.[23] Providers will need to consciously ask the child to answer first and encourage this by addressing the patient directly, having the child move to sit closer, making eye contact with the child, and finding ways to engage if the patients are distracted by electronics. Questions such as the frequency of abdominal pain or bleeding may seem straightforward to adults, but adolescents may need practice to anticipate them and have answers. Parents can be taught to play the role of coach and help the child think through responses before the clinic visit. The importance of having time alone with the provider has been emphasized repeatedly, and this can help parents also recognize the need for the patient to communicate well. Ideally this starts during midadolescence and gradually increases. Having patients voice their opinions regarding the plan is a step toward shared decision-making.

Communication beyond the clinic visit is a key component to adequate access to the health care system; this includes numerous types of communication, such as calling to report symptoms or for laboratory results. Although many patients with IBD feel most readily equipped at time of transition to talk to providers, their self-reported weakest skill is making and keeping appointments.[24] If a patient is experiencing new symptoms or signs of an IBD flare, knowing the channels of communication to their provider can prevent unnecessary emergency room utilization and delays in care. Additional factors come into play if patients are abroad or at a distance; they would need to bring their medications, determine how to get refills, and who to communicate with if they develop symptoms away from their primary gastroenterologist.

Providers have an obligation to guide and encourage the development of increasing self-management responsibility.[21] It is common for both patients and families to resist the early initiation of skill building, feeling this requirement is premature. However, although each task may be small, the process of learning and practicing each skill takes time. Mastery is best done when the adolescent is still home and not distracted by moving to a new apartment, college, or a new job. However, providers should have structure or embedded reminders because data demonstrate provider awareness of transition topics alone does not improve self-reported transition readiness skills in adolescent patients.25

The construct of self-management refers to a conceptual model of the interaction of health behaviors and related processes that patients and families engage in to care for a chronic condition.[26] Influences on self-management can be broken into different domains, including the individual, family, community, and health care system. Within each domain, there are modifiable and nonmodifiable factors. For example, in individuals their age, developmental level, race, and gender may be nonmodifiable, whereas their disease knowledge, ability to communicate symptoms, and coping style are modifiable. The goal of facilitating a successful transition involves intervening on modifiable factors in the context of what is fixed in each individual patient.

Modifiable factors such as health literacy, problem-solving ability, and social isolation are some risk factors that have been explored. Although transition can be difficult for all patients with IBD, additional ecological factors such as lower socioeconomic status and language barriers can be further obstacles in the process.[27] Public insurance, mental health concerns, active disease, and poor adherence seem to put patients with IBD at higher risk for poor transition outcomes.[28] Social support has been positively related to improved self-management and adherence to treatment in youth with IBD. For this age group, a sense of community within one's peer group can be especially meaningful, and in the United States and Canada events such as Camp Oasis and Camp Got2Go help provide a space to connect with others facing similar challenges.[29,30]

One self-management strategy includes coping skills training, which can enhance patient empowerment and perception of disease.[15] Another is to provide problem-solving skills training (PSST), which is a widely used method of improving self-efficacy in patients.[15] It involves teaching systematic ways of identifying barriers to self-management and helping to generate and implement structured solutions to such barriers. For example, a common self-management deficit is medication adherence in adolescents, and PSST may be able to help identify it as a problem, set up a plan such as setting daily alarms to address the deficit, and evaluate how successful the intervention is.

Ideally pediatric providers have been providing education and transition planning consistently since early adolescence, which is one meaning for the term "structured transition." However, the term also includes the concept of having special programming in the final 1 to 2 years before transfer. Structured transition programs have been shown to lead to significantly improved disease outcomes, especially in adherence to care and utilization of ambulatory care, with minimal economic impact.[10,31] Recent consensus guidelines recommend that all adolescents and young adults with pediatric-onset IBD should attend a structured transition program.[32] Models that have been studied included hybrid telehealth programs and hiring a transition coordinator for one-time transition interventions, both of which improved acquisition of self-management skills.[33–35] Another study in Germany looked at group patient education programs focused on transition skills comparing patients with IBD with patients who had diabetes.[36] The program enhanced the skills for self-management and transition, as well as demonstrated increased quality of life measures.

ASSESSING READINESS

Readiness has been thought to be a prerequisite for initiation of transfer for many providers. Assessment of readiness to transition is difficult to measure, as there has not been a uniform definition of transition success, but providers do agree on many of the components.[37]

Different assessment tools have been used to assess readiness (**Table 1**).[44] Disease-specific assessments may be more tailored to the condition, but the generalized tools are popular and can be used in those patients with more than one disease process or health issue.

The transition readiness assessment questionnaire (TRAQ) is one of the most widely used tools to assess transition readiness, being validated and applicable for all medical conditions.[38] Domains covered include managing medications, keeping appointments, talking with providers, and following health issues. Other assessment forms may have more or less domains but typically cover very similar topics. The TRAQ answers are deliberately modeled on the stages of change: precontemplation, contemplation, initiation, action, and mastery.[45] This language is common for many of the assessment tools.

Even with validated tools such as this, there is no agreement on what the threshold should be for a patient to achieve before being deemed ready for transition.[46] At one institution that set an internal benchmark of 90% by expert opinion, only 5.6% of older

Table 1
Readiness assessment tools

	Validated?	Disease: Specific vs General	Number of Items	Type of Answers	Administered by
TRAQ[38]	Yes	General	20 items	5 pt Likert	Self
TRxANSITION[39]	Yes	General	32 items	Open-ended Graded 0–1	Trained provider
STARx[40]	Yes	General	18 items	4 pt Likert	Self
RAISE[41]	Yes	General	—	Open-ended	Trained examiner
ICN Self-Management Handbook Transition Checklist[42]	No	IBD	21 items	3 pt Likert	Self
NASPGHAN IBD Checklist[43]	No	IBD	4–10 items per age	Yes/no	Patient and provider

adolescents and young adults met such a goal.[21] Although such a benchmark may be a hopeful goal to strive for, it does not set realistic expectations for transition or health care management in adulthood, as studies have shown adults with IBD fall short of this metric.[47] The self-report style of assessment is prone to overreporting of skills, as was shown recently with a study assessing the validity of a transition checklist compared with a skills-based practicum.[45]

The TRxANSITION Scale is another well-known tool. In this assessment, a trained researcher asks open-ended questions of the patient and then scores the response with 1 for complete answer, 0.5 for partially correct, and 0 for incorrect or does not know.[39] There are 10 domains. The nature of the questions allows for deeper understanding of the patient's skills and knowledge. However, providing and training the assessors does consume resources.

A shorter self-survey version was created and validated, called the STARx questionnaire. It has 18 questions with 4-point Likert scored answers.[40]

The RAISE (Readiness Assessment of Independence for Specialty Encounter) tool was developed to help assess readiness and self-management with all chronic conditions.[41] It is unique in its developmental breadth, starting from diagnosis of conditions that can be as early as birth, allowing for consistent and developmentally appropriate education. As opposed to other tools that are patient questionnaire–based, the RAISE acts as a guideline tool for providers and also includes psychosocial barriers to consider that may impede on the mastery of skills.

Some assessments focus on a specific modifiable factor, such as the IBD Yourself questionnaire, which looks at self-efficacy in adolescents with IBD. Self-efficacy is one's belief in themselves to organize and enact actions to handle prospective situations.[48]

There are unique considerations for patients with cognitive delay, as some patients will require significant support from parents and caregivers.[49] Guardianship is considered for patients who will need others to control financial, medical, and personal decisions. Pediatric patients with disabilities will often age out of the system at age 22 years. Patients may have the capacity for autonomy in some areas and need assistance in others. Medical decisions are more likely to need oversight due to the severity of consequences.

TRANSFER

The penultimate step to transfer is setting up an appointment to establish care with an adult gastroenterologist. Starting the discussion of choosing an adult provider should depend on the realities of how quickly care can be established on the adult side, but generally consider starting the conversation 6 to 9 months before anticipated transition.[49] Assess the patient's planned location for the following years, which may be affected by moving or college. Doc4me (doc4me-app.com) is a phone app developed by NASPGHAN to help patients find adult IBD providers in a specific area. This app can be helpful for both the initial transition from pediatric care, as well as any further transfers of care.[50] A resource such as this one can help boost a patient's confidence about finding other providers in the future.

As the time for transfer approaches, it is beneficial to acknowledge that strong emotions are often involved in the transition process from patient, parent, and provider, which can make the process more difficult. These emotional barriers may impede the transition process, which includes patient and family aversion to losing a bond with a trusted provider and fear of change, as well as pediatric gastroenterologist concern for transfer of care to someone who may know the patient and their history less well. Loyalty to the pediatric gastroenterologist-patient relationship, or concern regarding the competency of the adult provider, can cause anxiety from all parties. This anxiety may lead parties to not bring up transition to avoid difficult emotions. A way to transform our perception of it is to reframe it into a graduation from pediatric care, focusing on it as a patient success and positive acknowledgment of growth.[16]

It can be very helpful to patients and families to explain that the culture of pediatric and adult-centered care differs[49] (**Table 2**). Endorsing that the shift in culture is age-appropriate and eventually appreciated by patients is important. The pediatric provider as a trusted authority, explaining differences they may see in the care after transfer, can mitigate resistance to the unfamiliar and prevent bounceback after initial transfer.[51]

There are models of transfer that vary throughout gastroenterology practices. Joint clinics, alternating adult and pediatric visits, patient navigators, warm handoffs, and patient passports or medical summaries have all been explored in the literature. Results reported are often based on observational studies or expert opinion. The realities of local practice, provider preference, payment models, and patient comorbidities affect the transfer options.

Joint clinics have been studied as a modality for more seamless transfer of care, allowing patients to meet their future provider, have a more gradual introduction to adult care, and experience implicit approval by their pediatric provider.[52] Thought should be given to which setting houses the clinic, as ancillary services will help reinforce the cultural milieu. Billing and time constraints may preclude this strategy in some regions. Similarly, alternating visits for a year may not be possible for insurance reasons and have the disadvantage of delayed cultural assimilation to the new provider.

Another method to improve transfer is the "warm handoff," involving in-person or virtual synchronous communication between pediatric and adult gastroenterologists, which may or may not have the patient and family present. Situations to consider a warm handoff include when a patient is known to be particularly stoic or an unreliable historian or if there are other considerations medically or socially that are best conveyed to the receiving provider in real-time. For many patients who have minimal complexity, a transfer summary may suffice.

The structure of an ideal transfer summary or passport is still evolving. But it is crucial to ensure the patient has a portable and accessible medical summary to facilitate smooth collaboration and transfer.[5] This portable summary can take many forms, such as a physical or electronic "IBD passport" and should include diagnosis, prior medications, relevant endoscopic and radiographic findings, past surgical history, and immunization history.[53] Some components are clearly needed such as diagnostic evaluation and previous treatments. However, other details may be considered necessary by some providers and excessive by others. Whether the receiving provider has access to the full medical records may influence what is included in the summary provided.

Table 2
Cultural differences in care

	Pediatric	Adult
Priority values	Nurturance, connection, and warmth	Autonomy, respect, and privacy
Centered on	Family	Individual
Model	Collaborative	Investigative
Patient should feel	Comfortable	Respected

Given the intricacies of the transfer step, the enlistment of a patient navigator for this process can be greatly beneficial.[54] A patient navigator at this stage would be able to assist with preparation, health system navigation, and could also provide posttransfer support to ensure a successful transition. However, the significant resources needed for a navigator may not be available.

In surveys regarding the transition process, logistical issues such as parking, physically finding the office, making appointments, and sending records were cited as the most difficult part.[55] Having the patient preview the location or do a practice run can be helpful. They may need to be reminded to call the new office to confirm their medical records arrived and to ask relatives to review family history details with them. Patients may know or bring lists of current and past medications, medication allergies, and past surgeries.

The final pediatric visit is often filled with emotion. However, it is important to provide closure logistically and emotionally. Using a checklist has been helpful for many providers. **Table 3** goes through past, present, and future as a way to organize the visit. Having the provider frame the transition and transfer as a positive step, a graduation, is beneficial for both the patient and family. It also helps to normalize the emotions felt by all stakeholders at this time.

The pediatric provider may not know if the transfer was successful and that the patient was able to make their appointment to establish care. Asking the patient to leave a message that the visit was accomplished helps to establish accountability for completing the visit. It is also useful to ensure no important information is missed. Communicating by phone or e-mail may give the pediatric provider a chance also to validate the patient experience. In case the patient does not reach out, ideally, the pediatric provider will know the date of that visit, so they have the option to reach out for acknowledgment from the adult gastroenterologist after the first visit.

Unless there are significant extenuating circumstances, a patient should not return to pediatric care after they have established care in the adult health care system. Although patients will often feel uncertain after their first appointment, the pediatric provider can provide reassurance and help normalize those feelings. If absolutely

Table 3 Last visit checklist	
Checking in	Make sure there are no new medical issues or major life events that could postpone the final visit
Review the Past	Review and summarize the patient's course Reminisce about how far the patient has come during your time together
Discuss the Present	Point out that this is a milestone, a graduation Talk about emotions (your own if possible) regarding sadness at the patient leaving but pride in the growth seen Express confidence that the patient will do well in the adult world
Preview the Future	Explain the cultural differences to be expected in adult medical care Enumerate the advantages of the adult provider (medical and social) Endorse the new provider but be honest about whether it is based on knowing the provider personally or by reputation Explain your interest in the patient continues and what are appropriate ways to remain in touch (cards or email) Detail who is in charge in the interval between this goodbye and the first adult visit (if they get sick or run out of medicines)
Final Gesture	Handshake or hug or other gesture

necessary such as a patient-provider mismatch, the pediatric provider can help them find a different adult gastroenterologist. If this is the case, the patient may need extra reassurance to confirm that the patient can indeed handle being in adult care and dispel any sense of failure for the mismatch.

ROLE OF ADULT PROVIDER

HCT has developed over time from a sole focus on the pediatric responsibility of facilitating a successful transition to a joint responsibility between pediatric and adult providers.[3] In addition to managing their disease process, there are other considerations for adult gastroenterologists that may further optimize a young adult's health outcome. For a patient emerging from a lifetime of pediatric care, they will likely be nervous on their first few visits, with half of the respondents in a survey describing their first visit as "terrifying."[55] Information given at that visit may not be retained well and should be repeated at other visits. Reassurance to patients can be very meaningful, as well as clearly set expectations and goals.[32] The main concern of young adult patients with IBD during the transition to adult care was meeting a new team and building new relationships.[56] In the first year of transfer, adult providers could consider planning more frequent visits with longer visit lengths to aid in transition and acclimation.[57]

When transferring to adult care, it can be unclear what the role of the parent or guardian should be. It is reasonable to invite them to the first visit to establish care, to both provide closure for them and also give them a chance to provide any additional history or context. Adolescents often do not have a strong grasp of family history, which is a place where parents can fill in the gaps. Past the first visit, encouraging the patient to come alone or take ownership of their visit and care is ideal.

It is important to recognize that patients with IBD may have delayed "adulting" skills. Negative consequences on psychosocial development are prevalent in adults with IBD, with findings showing lower rates of employment and higher rates of social isolation among this population.[58] Understanding the time scale of the emerging adult and the delays caused by medical illness can help adult providers estimate more appropriate expectations for patients transitioning into their practice. More than 40% of adults with IBD between the ages of 25 to 50 years report not being fully independent in their health maintenance tasks; therefore, patient education and advocacy does not stop after transition, and patients would benefit from longitudinal support in developing skills for self-management.[47]

SUMMARY

The gradual and intentional movement of pediatric patients toward medical self-management has been endorsed as important by many professional societies. This process should start in early adolescence and can use various task lists to help establish expectations for the development of skills by the patient. Age or developmental milestones or readiness can be used as a criterion for transfer to adult care; however, anticipatory reminders will be more difficult to plan if the latter is used. Readiness can be assessed through self-report through various tools or assessed through a trained provider. These reported skills may not fully match what can be found through practical skill assessment.

Questions remain regarding the best transfer criteria, optimal timing, and ideal handoff strategies. Even the outcome of successful transitioning is not well defined and thus can be hard to track. The momentum toward quality transition care grows, among individual practitioners and multicenter organizations alike. Collaborations such as the ImproveCareNow network will collect larger aggregates of data to better understand patient needs and factors that affect outcomes.[59] Identifying which sets of patients require which strategies to improve self-management and have successful collaboration with adult medical providers will focus on transition care efforts. Patients with well-planned transitions seem to have improved health and outcomes for their IBD.

The interest in transition care has led to a focus on patient factors beyond medical regimens. The skills, self-efficacy, problem-solving, and confidence gained by pediatric patients in the process will have profound positive consequences during the emerging adult years and perhaps beyond. Searching for how to best teach and empower patients and families will gradually become more patient-specific as understanding of the process evolves. Meanwhile, the publication of literature with observations and studies can help in a very practical way.

CLINICS CARE POINTS

- Approximately 25% of patients with IBD will be diagnosed before age 20 years. Given they are likely to have more complex and severe disease, these children will need ongoing care into adult years, ideally in a seamless fashion.

- There is discordance among health care providers about when the transition process should take place and what should be triggers or indications to require transfer. Ideally, the timing is defined in a way that can be anticipated and discussed for several years before the transfer. Anticipation and planning can improve the chances for a smooth and successful transfer of care.

- Transition task lists can be helpful to quickly assess developmentally appropriate topics and set expectations for behaviors. Integration of transition tools into electronic health records has been shown as an effective way to standardize and distribute self-assessments and skills practicums during patient visits, without significantly affecting clinical workflow.

- Models of transfer vary throughout gastroenterology practices. Joint clinics, alternating adult and pediatric visits, patient navigators, warm handoffs, and patient passports or medical summaries have all been explored previously. The realities of local practice, provider preference, payment models, and patient comorbidities affect the transfer options.

DISCLOSURE

The authors have nothing to disclose.

REFERENCES

1. Chu PY, Maslow GR, von Isenburg M, et al. Systematic review of the impact of transition interventions for adolescents with chronic illness on transfer from pediatric to adult healthcare. J Pediatr Nurs 2015;30(5):e19–27.
2. Zhao X, Bjerre LM, Nguyen GC, et al. Health Services Use during Transition from Pediatric to Adult Care for Inflammatory Bowel Disease: A Population-Based Study Using Health Administrative Data. J Pediatr 2018;203:280–7.e4.
3. White PH, Cooley WC. Supporting the Health Care Transition From Adolescence to Adulthood in the Medical Home. Pediatrics 2018;142(5):20.
4. GotTransition.org, "GotTransition® - Six Core Elements of Health Care TransitionTM," GotTransition.org. Available at: https://www.gottransition.org/six-core-elements/. Accessed October 06, 2022.
5. Rosen DS, Blum RW, Britto M, et al. Transition to adult health care for adolescents and young adults with chronic conditions. J Adolesc Health 2003;33(4):309–11.

6. Rosen MJ, Dhawan A, Saeed SA. Inflammatory Bowel Disease in Children and Adolescents. Arch Pediatr Adolesc Med 2015;169(11):1053.

7. Kern I, Schoffer O, Richter T, et al. Current and projected incidence trends of pediatric-onset inflammatory bowel disease in Germany based on the Saxon Pediatric IBD Registry 2000–2014 –a 15-year evaluation of trends, *PLoS One*, 17 (9), 2022, e0274117.

8. Knudsen MM, Jakobsen C, Vester-Andersen MK, et al. Paediatric onset inflammatory bowel disease is a distinct and aggressive phenotype—a comparative population-based study. GastroHep 2019;1(6):266–73.

9. Mollah T, Lee D, Giles E. Impact of a new young adult inflammatory bowel disease transition clinic on patient satisfaction and clinical outcomes. J Paediatr Child Health 2022;58(6):1053–9.

10. McCartney S, Lindsay JO, Russell RK, et al. Benefits of Structured Pediatric to Adult Transition in Inflammatory Bowel Disease, *J Pediatr Gastroenterol Nutr,* 74 (2), 2022, 208–214.

11. Cole R, Ashok D, Razack A, et al. Evaluation of Outcomes in Adolescent Inflammatory Bowel Disease Patients Following Transfer From Pediatric to Adult Health Care Services: Case for Transition. J Adolesc Health 2015;57(2):212–7.

12. S. M. Fernandes et al., "Clinician perceptions of transition of patients with pediatric-onset chronic disease to adult medical care: Comparing a pediatric facility integrated within an adult institution with a free-standing pediatric hospital," p. 1.

13. Bensen R, McKenzie RB, Fernandes SM, et al. Transitions in Pediatric Gastroenterology: Results of a National Provider Survey. J Pediatr Gastroenterol Nutr 2016; 63(5):488–93.

14. Huang JS, Yueh R, Wood K, et al. Harnessing the Electronic Health Record to Distribute Transition Services to Adolescents With Inflammatory Bowel Disease, *J Pediatr Gastroenterol Nutr,* 70 (2), 2020, 200–204.

15. Plevinsky J, Greenley R, Fishman L. Self-management in patients with inflammatory bowel disease: strategies, outcomes, and integration into clinical care. Clin Exp Gastroenterol 2016;9:259–67.

16. "Putting the Good in Goodbye: The Pediatrician's Role in Framing a Positive Transition to Adult Care." Available at: https://journals-sagepub-com.ezproxy.bu.edu/doi/epub/10.1177/00099228221102711. Accessed September 22, 2022.

17. van Gaalen MAC, van Pieterson M, van den Brink G, et al. Rotterdam Transition Test: A Valid Tool for Monitoring Disease Knowledge in Adolescents With Inflammatory Bowel Disease, *J Pediatr Gastroenterol Nutr,* 74 (1), 2022, 60–67.

18. Vaz KKH, Carmody JK, Zhang Y, et al. Evaluation of a Novel Educational Tool in Adolescents With Inflammatory Bowel Disease: The NEAT Study. J Pediatr Gastroenterol Nutr 2019;69(5):564–9.

19. Gumidyala AP, Plevinsky JM, Poulopoulos N, et al. What Teens Do Not Know Can Hurt Them: An Assessment of Disease Knowledge in Adolescents and Young Adults with IBD. Inflamm Bowel Dis 2017;23(1):89–96.

20. Benchimol EJ, Walters TD, Kaufman M, et al. Assessment of knowledge in adolescents with inflammatory bowel disease using a novel transition tool. Inflamm Bowel Dis 2011;17(5):1131–7.

21. Gray WN, Holbrook E, Morgan PJ, et al. Transition Readiness Skills Acquisition in Adolescents and Young Adults with Inflammatory Bowel Disease: Findings from Integrating Assessment into Clinical Practice. Inflamm Bowel Dis 2015;21(5): 1125–31.

22. Crume B, Mitchell PD, Fishman LN. Infusion appointment self-management among adolescents with inflammatory bowel disease. J Pediatr Gastroenterol Nutr 2022. https://doi.org/10.1097/MPG.0000000000003678.

23. van Groningen J, Ziniel S, Arnold J, et al. When independent healthcare behaviors develop in adolescents with inflammatory bowel disease. Inflamm Bowel Dis 2012;18(12):2310–4.

24. Arvanitis M, Hart LC, DeWalt DA, et al. Transition Readiness Not Associated With Measures of Health in Youth With IBD, Inflamm Bowel Dis, 27 (1), 2020, 49–57.

25. Fishman LN, Ziniel SI, Adrichem ME, et al. Provider Awareness Alone Does Not Improve Transition Readiness Skills in Adolescent Patients With Inflammatory Bowel Disease. J Pediatr Gastroenterol Nutr 2014;59(2):221–4.

26. Modi AC, Pai AL, Hommel KA, et al. Pediatric Self-management: A Framework for Research, Practice, and Policy, Pediatrics, 129 (2), 2012, e473–e485.

27. Javalkar K, Johnson M, Kshirsagar AV, et al. Ecological Factors Predict Transition Readiness/Self-Management in Youth With Chronic Conditions. J Adolesc Health 2016;58(1):40–6.

28. Pearlstein H, Bricker J, Michel HK, et al. Predicting Suboptimal Transitions in Adolescents With Inflammatory Bowel Disease. J Pediatr Gastroenterol Nutr 2021; 72(4):563–8.

29. "Camp Oasis | Crohn's & Colitis Foundation." Available at: https://www.crohn scolitisfoundation.org/get-involved/camp-oasis. Accessed November 01, 2022.

30. "Camp Got2Go - Camp Got2Go - Crohn's and Colitis Canada." Available at: https://crohnsandcolitis.ca/Support-for-You/Summer-camp. Accessed November 01, 2022.

31. Gabriel P, McManus M, Rogers K, et al. Outcome Evidence for Structured Pediatric to Adult Health Care Transition Interventions: A Systematic Review. J Pediatr 2017;188:263–9.e15.

32. Fu N, Bollegala N, Jacobson K, et al. Canadian Consensus Statements on the Transition of Adolescents and Young Adults with Inflammatory Bowel Disease from Pediatric to Adult Care: A Collaborative Initiative Between the Canadian IBD Transition Network and Crohn's and Colitis Canada, J Can Assoc Gastroenterol, 5 (3), 2022, 105–115.

33. Gray WN, Wagoner ST, Schaefer MR, et al. Transition to Adult IBD Care: A Pilot Multi-Site, Telehealth Hybrid Intervention, J Pediatr Psychol, 46 (1), 2021, 1–11.

34. Gray WN, Holbrook E, Dykes D, et al. Improving IBD Transition, Self-management, and Disease Outcomes With an In-clinic Transition Coordinator. J Pediatr Gastroenterol Nutr 2019;69(2):194–9.

35. Waschmann M, Lin HC, Stellway JE. 'Adulting' with IBD: Efficacy of a Novel Virtual Transition Workshop for Pediatric Inflammatory Bowel Disease. J Pediatr Nurs 2021;60:223–9.

36. Schmidt S, Markwart H, Bomba F, et al. Differential effect of a patient-education transition intervention in adolescents with IBD vs. diabetes, Eur J Pediatr, 177 (4), 2018, 497–505.

37. Bihari A, Olayinka L, Kroeker KI. "Outcomes in Patients with Inflammatory Bowel Disease Transitioning from Pediatric to Adult Care: A Scoping Review. J Pediatr Gastroenterol Nutr 2022. https://doi.org/10.1097/MPG.0000000000003581.

38. Sawicki GS, Lukens-Bull K, Yin X, et al. Measuring the Transition Readiness of Youth with Special Healthcare Needs: Validation of the TRAQ—Transition Readiness Assessment Questionnaire. J Pediatr Psychol 2011;36(2):160–71.

39. "A Clinical Tool to Measure the Components of Health-Care Transition from Pediatric Care to Adult Care: The UNC TRxANSITION Scale." Available at: https://www.

tandfonline.com/doi/epdf/10.3109/0886022X.2012.678171?needAccess=true& role=button. Accessed December 22, 2022.

40. Cohen SE, Hooper SR, Javalkar K, et al. Self-Management and Transition Readiness Assessment: Concurrent, Predictive and Discriminant Validation of the STARx Questionnaire, *J Pediatr Nurs*, 30 (5), 2015, 668–676.

41. Shanske S, Bond J, Ross A, et al. Validation of the RAISE (Readiness Assessment of Independence for Specialty Encounters) Tool: Provider-Based Transition Evaluation. J Pediatr Nurs 2021;59:103–9.

42. ImproveCareNowTM, "Self-Management Handbook," ImproveCareNow. Available at: https://www.improvecarenow.org/handbook. Accessed December 22, 2022.

43. "NASPGHAN - Inflammatory Bowel Disease," NASPGHAN. Available at: https://naspghan.org/professional-resources/medical-professional-resources/inflammatory-bowel-disease/. Accessed December 22, 2022.

44. de Silva PSA, Fishman LN. Transition of the patient with IBD from pediatric to adult care-an assessment of current evidence. Inflamm Bowel Dis 2014;20(8): 1458–64.

45. Huang JS, Cruz R, Kruth R, et al. Evaluating transition readiness: Is self-report valid as the gold standard? J Pediatr Gastroenterol Nutr 2023. https://doi.org/10.1097/MPG.0000000000003680.

46. Huang JS, Tobin A, Tompane T. Clinicians Poorly Assess Health Literacy–Related Readiness for Transition to Adult Care in Adolescents With Inflammatory Bowel Disease. Clin Gastroenterol Hepatol 2012;10(6):626–32.

47. Fishman LN, Mitchell PD, Lakin PR, et al. Are expectations too high for transitioning adolescents with IBD? Examining adult medication knowledge and self-management skills. J Pediatr Gastroenterol Nutr 2016;63(5):494–9.

48. Zijlstra M, De Bie C, Breij L, et al. Self-efficacy in adolescents with inflammatory bowel disease: A pilot study of the 'IBD-yourself', a disease-specific questionnaire. J. Crohns Colitis 2013;7(9):e375–85.

49. L. N. Fishman, Are Your Pediatric Patients Ready for Adult Health Care? What to Do and How to Do It. Nova Science Publishers, Inc, 2015. Accessed: Aug. 19, 2022. Online. Available at: https://novapublishers.com/shop/are-your-pediatric-patients-ready-for-adult-health-care-what-to-do-and-how-to-do-it/.

50. "Home," Doc4me. Available at: https://www.doc4me-app.com/. Accessed September 29, 2022.

51. Huang JS, Gottschalk M, Pian M, et al. Transition to Adult Care: Systematic Assessment of Adolescents with Chronic Illnesses and their Medical Teams. J Pediatr 2011;159(6):994–8.e2.

52. Davis AM, Brown RF, Taylor JL, et al. Transition Care for Children With Special Health Care Needs. Pediatrics 2014;134(5):900, 908.

53. Muhammad R, Law TL, Limdi JK. The IBD passport: Bridging another gap in quality of care? J. Crohns Colitis 2012;6(2):261–2.

54. Dimitropoulos G, Morgan-Maver E, Allemang B, et al. Health care stakeholder perspectives regarding the role of a patient navigator during transition to adult care. BMC Health Serv Res 2019;19:390.

55. Plevinsky JM, Gumidyala AP, Fishman LN. Transition experience of young adults with inflammatory bowel diseases (IBD): a mixed methods study: Transition experience of young adults with IBD. Child Care Health Dev 2015;41(5):755–61.

56. Karim S, Porter JA, McCombie A, et al. Transition clinics: an observational study of themes important to young people with inflammatory bowel disease. Transl Pediatr 2019;8(1):839–89.

57. Jawaid N, Jeyalingam T, Nguyen G, et al. Paediatric to Adult Transition of Care in IBD: Understanding the Current Standard of Care Among Canadian Adult Academic Gastroenterologists. J Can Assoc Gastroenterol 2019;gwz023. https://doi.org/10.1093/jcag/gwz023.
58. Hummel TZ, Tak E, Maurice-Stam H, et al. Psychosocial Developmental Trajectory of Adolescents With Inflammatory Bowel Disease. J Pediatr Gastroenterol Nutr 2013;57(2):219–24.
59. ImproveCareNowTM, "Purpose & Success," ImproveCareNow. Available at: https://www.improvecarenow.org/purpose-success. Accessed September 29, 2022.

Moving?

Make sure your subscription moves with you!

To notify us of your new address, find your **Clinics Account Number** (located on your mailing label above your name), and contact customer service at:

Email: journalscustomerservice-usa@elsevier.com

800-654-2452 (subscribers in the U.S. & Canada)
314-447-8871 (subscribers outside of the U.S. & Canada)

Fax number: 314-447-8029

Elsevier Health Sciences Division
Subscription Customer Service
3251 Riverport Lane
Maryland Heights, MO 63043

*To ensure uninterrupted delivery of your subscription, please notify us at least 4 weeks in advance of move.

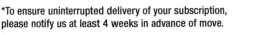